Liam Moore

The Essence of the Holistic Mind
A Deep Dive into the Unity of Existence

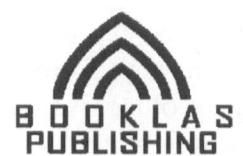

Original Title: The Essence of the Holistic Mind
Copyright © 2025, published by Luiz Antonio dos Santos ME.

This book is a non-fiction work exploring practices and concepts in the field of holism and interconnectedness. Through a comprehensive approach, the author offers insights into philosophy, ecology, quantum science, and spirituality, promoting an integrated vision of reality and personal transformation.

1st Edition
Production Team
Author: Liam Moore
Editor: Luiz Santos
Cover Design: Studios Booklas/ Sophie Williams
Layout Design: Jonathan Reed

Publication and Identification
The Essence of the Holistic Mind
Booklas, 2025
Categories: Philosophy / Spirituality / Holism
DDC: 128.2 - CDU: 141.3
All rights reserved to:
Luiz Antonio dos Santos ME / Booklas

No part of this book may be reproduced, stored in a retrieval system, or transmitted in any form—electronic, mechanical, photocopying, recording, or otherwise—without prior and express authorization from the copyright holder.

Summary

Systematic Index 5
Prologue 8
Chapter 1 An Integrated View of the World 11
Chapter 2 From Ancient Origins to Modernity 17
Chapter 3 Connections Between the Whole and the Parts 25
Chapter 4 Quantum Physics, Biology and Ecology 33
Chapter 5 The Quest for Unity 40
Chapter 6 The Gaia Hypothesis 48
Chapter 7 Respecting the Interconnectedness of Life 56
Chapter 8 Holism and Sustainability 64
Chapter 9 The Wisdom of Ecosystems 73
Chapter 10 Addressing Global Challenges 82
Chapter 11 The Holistic Mind 91
Chapter 12 Medicina Holística e Bem-Estar 99
Chapter 13 Forming Complete Human Beings 107
Chapter 14 Expressions of Totality 115
Chapter 15 Living in Harmony 123
Chapter 16 Beyond Material Growth 130
Chapter 17 Systemic Visions for a Better World 139
Chapter 18 Ferramentas para a Integração 149
Chapter 19 Celebrating Unity in Plurality 158
Chapter 20 Building an Inclusive World 167
Chapter 21 Holistic Utopias and Dystopias 176
Chapter 22 Converging Towards a New Reality 185

Chapter 23 Global Transformation 193
Chapter 24 The Search for the Meaning of Life 199
Chapter 25 Living Holism in Daily Life 208
Epilogue 218

Systematic Index

Chapter 1: An Integrated View of the World - This chapter explores the contrast between the modern reductionist paradigm and the holistic view of the world.

Chapter 2: From Ancient Origins to Modernity - Discusses the history of holistic thinking from ancient times to the present day.

Chapter 3: Connections Between the Whole and the Parts - Explores the relationship between the whole and the parts in different philosophical traditions.

Chapter 4: Quantum Physics, Biology and Ecology - Examines how contemporary science reveals a deeply interconnected reality.

Chapter 5: The Quest for Unity - Discusses spirituality and the search for understanding the essential unity that permeates all existence.

Chapter 6: The Gaia Hypothesis - Explores the Gaia Hypothesis, which presents Earth as a self-regulating living organism.

Chapter 7: Respecting the Interconnectedness of Life - Discusses deep ecology and the understanding of the interconnectedness between all life forms on the planet.

Chapter 8: Holism and Sustainability - Examines the pursuit of a sustainable future and the need for a holistic approach.

Chapter 9: The Wisdom of Ecosystems - Explores how nature operates as a large, dynamic, interconnected system that maintains ecological balance.

Chapter 10: Addressing Global Challenges - Discusses the climate crisis and the need for a holistic approach to address global challenges.

Chapter 11: The Holistic Mind - Explores the human mind as a dynamic field of interactions between body, emotions, thoughts, and subtle dimensions of existence.

Chapter 12: Holistic Medicine and Well-being - Discusses human health and the holistic approach to medicine and well-being.

Chapter 13: Forming Complete Human Beings - Examines education as a transformative process that goes beyond the mere transmission of information.

Chapter 14: Expressions of Totality - Explores art and creativity as essential manifestations of human experience.

Chapter 15: Living in Harmony - Discusses human connection and its influence on our emotional, mental, and physical health.

Chapter 16: Beyond Material Growth - Examines contemporary economics and the need for a new economic paradigm that considers human well-being and environmental sustainability.

Chapter 17: Systemic Visions for a Better World - Discusses modern societies and the need for political approaches that transcend fragmentation and immediate interests.

Chapter 18: Tools for Integration - Explores the rapid evolution of technology and innovation and the need for a holistic approach to these tools.

Chapter 19: Celebrating Unity in Plurality - Discusses cultural diversity and the importance of valuing and celebrating it.

Chapter 20: Building an Inclusive World - Examines the pursuit of social justice and equity as fundamental cornerstones for building more harmonious societies.

Chapter 21: Holistic Utopias and Dystopias - Explores conceptions of the future and the importance of a holistic approach in shaping these projections.

Chapter 22: Converging Towards a New Reality - Discusses the understanding of reality and the potential convergence between science and spirituality.

Chapter 23: Global Transformation - Examines the process of global transformation and the role of individuals in building a more balanced and sustainable future.

Chapter 24: The Search for the Meaning of Life - Discusses the search for the meaning of life as an intrinsic journey to the human experience.

Chapter 25: Living Holism in Daily Life - Explores what it means to live holistically and how to adopt this perspective in everyday life.

Prologue

By Luiz Santos, Editor

There are books that inform, books that inspire, and books that transform. What you now hold in your hands is not merely a book—it is a passage, an invitation to rediscover a way of seeing the world that has long been forgotten, buried beneath the layers of modern distractions. If you allow it, these pages will dissolve the illusions of separation, unveiling a reality far greater than what conventional thought has led us to believe.

We live in an age of fragmentation, where knowledge is divided into disciplines, where humanity perceives itself as detached from nature, where the mind is often considered separate from the body, and the spirit dismissed as an abstraction. Yet, beneath this illusion of division lies a truth as old as existence itself: all things are interconnected. Every action, every thought, every breath is part of an intricate web that binds the seen and the unseen, the material and the immaterial, the self and the cosmos.

This book is not here to impose doctrines, nor to provide simple answers to complex questions. Instead, it is a key—one that unlocks doors you may not have known existed. It guides you through the history of holistic thought, from ancient traditions that understood the sacred harmony of existence to modern scientific discoveries that confirm what sages have long intuited: that consciousness, nature, and reality itself are not separate entities but expressions of a single, unified field of being.

As you immerse yourself in these pages, you will encounter ideas that may challenge you, perspectives that may unsettle you, and insights that may profoundly shift the way you relate to the world. You will see how quantum physics, biology, ecology, and philosophy converge, revealing patterns of unity within what once seemed chaotic. You will explore how indigenous wisdom, mystical traditions, and contemporary science echo the same fundamental truth: that separation is an illusion, and wholeness is the ultimate reality.

I have had the privilege of reading this work before it reaches you, and I can assure you—this is not a book that you will simply read and set aside. It is a book that will linger in your thoughts, that will whisper to you in quiet moments, that will urge you to reconsider what you know and how you live. It will challenge the way you perceive the world, and if you are willing, it will change you.

But transformation requires openness. It requires the courage to question what you have been taught and the willingness to embrace a deeper truth. If you feel that call—if something in you stirs at the thought that reality may be more connected, more profound, more wondrous than you have been led to believe—then you are exactly where you need to be.

This journey is not about accumulating knowledge; it is about awakening wisdom. The pages ahead will not tell you what to think—they will show you how to see. They will not give you rigid conclusions—they will offer you new ways to perceive, to understand, to experience.

So take a breath. Set aside preconceived notions. Allow yourself to step into a different way of thinking, a different way of being. Let the words on these pages guide you, not as rules, but as stepping stones toward a greater understanding of yourself and the universe.

Are you ready?

Then turn the page. The journey begins now.

Chapter 1
An Integrated View of the World

The fragmentation of Western thought has its roots in the development of modern science, which, over the centuries, has built detailed knowledge about specific aspects of reality, but often at the expense of understanding the whole. This tendency can be observed in various areas of knowledge, from biology, which often studies organisms in isolation without considering their ecosystems, to economics, which analyzes financial indicators without taking into account the environmental and social impacts of productive activities. However, the deepening of this reductionist model has led to adverse consequences, such as ecological crises, social inequalities, and a growing sense of disconnection between individuals and the world around them. The need for a more integrated vision arises, therefore, as an essential counterpoint to balance this paradigm, promoting an understanding that values both the details and the relationships between them. This change of perspective does not imply the abandonment of the analytical method, but rather the complementation of this with a systemic approach, which allows us to see the fundamental interdependence between the various aspects of reality.

Adopting a holistic view does not only mean modifying the way we interpret the world, but also transforming the way we act within it. The perception of interconnectivity leads us to an expanded responsibility, as we understand that each individual choice has repercussions in a chain of events that goes beyond our immediate experience. Caring for the environment, for example, is not just an ecological issue, but also a decision that affects the health, economy, and quality of life of future generations. Similarly, the search for emotional and mental balance is not an isolated process, but something that is reflected in interpersonal relationships and in the social dynamics as a whole. By integrating this awareness into our daily decisions, we become agents of transformation, promoting a culture based on cooperation, mutual respect, and harmony among the various elements that make up life. This perspective not only enriches our understanding of reality, but also invites us to actively participate in the construction of a more sustainable and balanced world.

The fragmentation of the modern world is reflected in almost every aspect of our lives, from the way we think to the way we organize our societies. We have become accustomed to categorizing reality into seemingly distinct opposites: mind and body, human and nature, individual and society. This division is not just a mental habit, but a profound reflection of the institutional structures that shape our knowledge and our interactions. Science, for example, traditionally segments the universe into isolated parts for study – atoms, cells, organisms, societies – often ignoring the connections and interdependencies between these elements. However, by prioritizing the study of the parts without considering the whole, we run the risk of losing the essential understanding of the interactions that give meaning and coherence to reality. It's like trying to understand a symphony by analyzing each note separately, without ever listening to the complete melody.

This reductionist approach, although it has allowed significant advances in science and technology, has also imposed limitations on our vision of the world. In the name of specialization, we have created increasingly fragmented disciplines and fields of knowledge, which has made it difficult to build a broad and integrated understanding of life. However, throughout the twentieth century, a counter-movement began to gain strength: holism, which emphasizes that the whole is greater than the sum of its parts. This idea is not new; many philosophical and spiritual traditions have already pointed to this interconnectivity. Taoism, for example, has always emphasized the harmony between opposites, while Buddhism proposes the interdependence of all things. Similarly, the ancestral knowledge of various indigenous cultures recognizes the inseparable relationship between humans, nature, and cosmos.

In modern science, holism has found an echo in several areas of knowledge. In quantum physics, for example, it was discovered that subatomic particles cannot be understood in isolation, as their states are intertwined with those of other particles, even over great distances. In ecology, it is understood that an ecosystem cannot be reduced to a simple sum of organisms, because the interaction between them is fundamental to its existence. In psychology, approaches have emerged that consider not only the individual aspects of the mind, but also the social and emotional contexts in which the individual is inserted.

Bringing this perspective to our daily lives means understanding that our actions have implications that go far beyond ourselves. For example, caring for the environment is not just an ecological attitude, but also a commitment to public health, to the quality of life of future generations, and to the balance of the economy itself. A polluted river, in addition to being an environmental problem, impacts the health of the people who depend on it, agricultural productivity, and even the economy of the cities around it. Similarly, cultivating healthy and balanced relationships not only benefits the individuals involved, but also strengthens the social fabric as a whole, promoting greater cooperation and collective well-being.

However, adopting a holistic view also presents challenges. How to integrate different areas of knowledge without falling into superficiality? How to balance individual needs with collective ones? How to maintain respect for traditions and, at the same time, embrace innovations? These questions require constant reflection and an open dialogue between different fields of knowledge. However, this approach also opens up new opportunities, allowing us to rethink our relationship with the world and with the people around us. Holism offers us a path to a more sustainable and harmonious future, in which every choice made takes into account not only the immediate impacts, but also its long-term repercussions.

By recognizing the interconnectivity of all things, we expand not only our intellectual understanding, but also our ability to act in a more conscious and effective way. This means adopting a posture that values both specialized knowledge and the systemic vision, seeking solutions that take into account multiple factors and consequences. Education, for example, can play a fundamental role in this process, promoting a learning that not only informs, but also teaches to think in an integrated way, connecting disciplines and encouraging a more comprehensive view of the world. Similarly, public policies that adopt this approach can generate more positive and lasting impacts, by considering the environmental, social, and economic aspects as parts of the same interdependent system.

More than a theoretical change, this integrated perspective requires a transformation in the attitudes and values that guide our daily choices. Empathy and collaboration become fundamental pillars for this new way of living, because the awareness of interdependence leads us to recognize that individual well-being can only be fully achieved when we also promote collective well-being. Small actions, such as responsible consumption, the encouragement of the circular economy, and active participation in communities and collaborative projects, become concrete expressions of this new paradigm. In this way, we stop being mere spectators of the world's changes and become active agents in the construction of a more balanced future.

By adopting this integrated vision, we begin to perceive that the world is not composed of isolated parts, but by a continuous flow of relationships that influence each other. This understanding does not mean eliminating the differences, but learning to see them as complementary, promoting a dynamic balance between specialization and totality, tradition and innovation, individuality and collectivity. Thus, instead of living trapped in the fragmentation that has characterized much of modern history, we can follow a path that harmonizes knowledge and wisdom, reason and intuition, science and humanity. This new way of perceiving and interacting with the world can be the first step towards a deeper transformation, capable of reconnecting us not only with nature and with others, but also with ourselves.

Chapter 2
From Ancient Origins to Modernity

Holistic thinking, far from being a recent concept, has its roots in the most ancient traditions of humanity. Since the first philosophical and religious records, different civilizations have perceived the existence of an invisible link that connects all things. This understanding emerged both from the observation of nature and from the need to interpret reality in a comprehensive way, overcoming fragmented views of the world. The understanding that existence is an integrated system, where each element influences and is influenced by the whole, permeates the most diverse cultures and systems of knowledge. This approach did not arise from a single geographical point or a single tradition, but manifested itself simultaneously in different parts of the planet, adapting to the cultural characteristics of each people. Thus, holism has crossed the centuries, influencing ways of thinking and practices that extend from ancient philosophy to the most advanced scientific discoveries.

In the civilizations of the East and the West, holism has expressed itself in distinct ways, but always guided by the idea of totality and interconnection. In the East, for example, philosophical-religious doctrines, such as Taoism and Buddhism, emphasized universal harmony and the interdependence between all forms of existence. The concept of the Tao as a unifying force and the symbol of Yin-Yang illustrate the complementary duality that maintains cosmic balance. Similarly, the Buddhist notion of "dependent origin" suggests that nothing exists in isolation, a conception that echoes the modern ecological and systemic view of the world. In the West, the pre-Socratics already sought to understand the unity behind the diversity of the universe. Heraclitus, when stating that "everything flows," introduced the idea of a world in constant transformation, where the parts can only be understood from the whole. Plato and Aristotle, each in their own way, also contributed to an integrated view of reality, recognizing the interrelationship between the different aspects of existence.

    This holistic conception, present in ancient cultures, was reconfigured throughout history, suffering periods of obscurity and resurgence. During the Middle Ages, mechanistic thought gained strength, reducing the world to a compartmentalized structure, where phenomena were analyzed separately. However, holism never completely disappeared. With the advances of modern science, especially quantum physics and systemic biology, the evidence of interconnectivity became undeniable. Quantum entanglement demonstrated that particles can influence each other even at great distances, challenging the Cartesian view of separation between the elements of the universe. In biology, the understanding of organisms as integrated systems and ecology as a study of natural interactions reinforced the importance of a broad look at life. In the field of psychology, approaches such as that of Carl Jung, with his concept of the collective unconscious, and humanistic psychology, with its emphasis on the integration of the being, demonstrate that holism also extends to the understanding of the mind and human behavior. Today, faced with global challenges that demand integrated solutions, the holistic vision resurfaces as a pressing need, offering paths to a more balanced and sustainable approach to reality.

The holistic conceptions of the world are not a recent invention. Since the dawn of civilization, different cultures have developed ways of perceiving reality as an integrated whole, where each element exists in relation to the other. In the East, for example, Taoism emerged in China around the sixth century BC, presenting a vision of the universe based on the Tao, an invisible universal force that permeates all things. The famous symbol of Yin-Yang expresses this idea of interconnection and balance, representing the complementary duality that structures existence—light and darkness, masculine and feminine, rest and movement, all coexisting and influencing each other.

Buddhism, in turn, introduced an essentially holistic concept: the principle of "dependent origin" or "interdependence." According to this view, nothing in the universe exists in isolation; everything that arises, arises in relation to something else. This directly resonates with the idea that the whole is greater than the sum of its parts, a fundamental principle of holistic thought.

In the West, the pre-Socratic philosophers already reflected on the underlying unity of the cosmos. Heraclitus, for example, coined the famous expression "panta rhei"—"everything flows"—suggesting that reality is a dynamic process in constant transformation, where nothing remains fixed and everything is interconnected. Plato, with his theory of ideas, believed that the physical world was an imperfect manifestation of a higher and interconnected reality, while Aristotle emphasized that understanding the whole was essential to understanding the parts.

Beyond the great philosophical and religious traditions, holism has always been present in indigenous cultures around the world. For many native peoples, the Earth is not just a physical space, but a living entity, a sacred mother who nurtures and sustains all beings. Among the Guarani, for example, there is the concept of "Land without evil," a representation of a world in balance and harmony, where human beings live in communion with nature. This holistic vision is reflected in the daily practices of these cultures, which have always emphasized the interdependence between humans, animals, plants and natural elements.

These ancestral traditions carry a fundamental wisdom that resonates deeply in our era, marked by environmental and social crises. The conception that the well-being of humanity is intrinsically linked to the health of the planet is an idea that proves to be more relevant than ever in the face of the ecological challenges we face.

Despite having been a predominant vision during Antiquity, holistic thought was progressively supplanted by mechanism during the Middle Ages and, later, by the Scientific Revolution. The universe came to be understood as a large machine composed of isolated and predictable parts, governed by immutable mathematical laws. However, in the twentieth century, with scientific advances, holism resurfaced with force, bringing new perspectives on the interconnectivity of the cosmos.

In physics, Albert Einstein's discoveries about relativity and advances in quantum mechanics transformed the deterministic view of the universe. The phenomenon of quantum entanglement, for example, revealed that subatomic particles can influence each other instantaneously, even when separated by great distances. This discovery challenged the traditional understanding of space and time and brought a new perspective on the fundamental interconnectivity of reality.

Biology has also undergone a revolution in this regard. The biologist Ludwig von Bertalanffy developed the Systems Theory, which demonstrated that organisms cannot be understood as mere sets of isolated parts, but as integrated systems, where each element plays a role in the balance of the whole. Ecology, in turn, showed that ecosystems function as complex networks of interactions, where all forms of life are interconnected in a dynamic cycle of mutual dependence.

Holistic thinking has also found space in philosophy and psychology. Philosophers like Alfred North Whitehead developed a processual view of the universe, arguing that reality is not composed of static objects, but of events and relationships in constant transformation. Ken Wilber, on the other hand, structured an approach called "integral theory," which seeks to synthesize different fields of knowledge within a unified model.

In psychology, Carl Jung made a significant contribution by introducing the concept of "collective unconscious," a deep layer of the psyche that connects all human beings through shared archetypes. This concept suggests that the human mind cannot be understood in an isolated way, but as part of a larger whole that transcends the individual. In addition, approaches such as humanistic psychology and transpersonal psychology have come to emphasize the integration between mind, body and spirit, proposing a model of well-being based on the balance between these aspects.

In the 21st century, holism becomes more relevant than ever. The world faces complex global challenges, such as climate change, biodiversity loss and social inequalities, problems that cannot be solved with fragmented approaches. Interdependence is an inescapable reality, and understanding phenomena systemically can help us find more effective solutions to these crises.

By adopting a holistic view, we come to recognize that all our actions have consequences that reverberate beyond ourselves. This understanding can guide more sustainable public policies, more responsible business practices, and a more conscious lifestyle, promoting a balance between material progress and collective well-being.

The trajectory of holistic thought, from its ancient roots to its resignification in modern science, teaches us a fundamental lesson: everything is interconnected. And, as we move towards the future, this integrated vision can help us build a more harmonious and sustainable world, where each part contributes to the balance of the whole.

The rediscovery of holism in contemporaneity is not just an intellectual trend, but a practical necessity in the face of the challenges we face. As technology advances and global interconnectivity intensifies, it becomes evident that complex problems cannot be solved in isolation. The climate crisis, for example, is not just an environmental issue, but also an economic, social and political one, requiring solutions that consider multiple dimensions simultaneously. Fragmented thinking, which once provided significant advances, is now insufficient to deal with the complexity of today's world, reinforcing the urgency of approaches that integrate different areas of knowledge.

In this context, disciplines such as deep ecology, regenerative economics and integrative medicine demonstrate how holism can be applied in practice, promoting solutions that respect the interdependence of systems. Economic models based on the circularity of resources, medical treatments that consider not only the physical body, but also the emotional and spiritual aspects of the patient, and public policies that address well-being in a broad way are examples of how this perspective is being incorporated into different fields. More than a theoretical concept, holism emerges as a paradigm capable of guiding more balanced and sustainable choices, both at the individual and collective levels.

Looking to the future, the continuity of this resignification will depend on our ability to overcome artificial divisions and see the world as a living, dynamic and interdependent organism. The ancestral wisdom that grounded holistic conceptions can, therefore, find new forms of expression in science and society, encouraging a more harmonious model of development. The challenge that arises is not only to understand this vision, but to apply it concretely, transforming the way we interact with the planet, with others and with ourselves.

Chapter 3
Connections Between the Whole and the Parts

The relationship between the whole and the parts constitutes a fundamental question in the history of human thought, reflecting in diverse philosophical traditions that sought to understand the interconnection between the elements of reality. Since the most ancient civilizations, the perception that nature, society, and knowledge itself form integrated systems has led to the development of conceptions that transcend the fragmented view of the world. The search to understand the functioning of this totality has driven debates about the nature of existence, the structure of reality, and the principles that govern the relationship between individuals and the universe.

Holistic thought emerged as a response to this restlessness, proposing that no entity can be fully understood in isolation, but only in its broader context. This approach, present from pre-Socratic philosophy to contemporary conceptions, has shaped the development of knowledge by suggesting that the complexity of the universe is not reduced to the sum of its parts, but is manifested in patterns of interdependence that structure all human experience.

The evolution of philosophical thought shows that the understanding of the world has always oscillated between reductionist and holistic perspectives. While some currents sought to analyze reality in an atomistic way, fragmenting it into distinct and isolated elements, others emphasized the need to see the universe as an interconnected whole. This conceptual tension generated profound debates about the essence of existence and influenced how different societies interpreted natural, political, and social phenomena. The holistic view, in turn, by highlighting the intrinsic connections between the components of the world, allowed the emergence of theories that value the interdependence and complementarity of phenomena. Thus, philosophy, since its origins, has been a fertile field for investigations that challenge simplistic notions and promote a more integrated view of reality.

The recognition of connections between the whole and the parts not only underpins several philosophical traditions but also offers a conceptual framework for understanding human relations, natural dynamics, and the ethical principles that govern life in society. The idea that each individual is part of a larger system has profound implications in multiple fields of knowledge, influencing everything from ethics and politics to science and spirituality. This understanding suggests that phenomena cannot be analyzed in isolation, as their characteristics emerge from the network of interactions that constitute them. Thus, throughout the history of thought, holism has revealed itself to be an essential approach to the construction of a broader and more sophisticated understanding of existence, inspiring reflections that remain relevant in contemporary times.

In ancient Greece, the idea of holism was already present in the reflections of thinkers like Heraclitus and Parmenides, who, although they had seemingly contrasting views, shared an interest in understanding reality as an interconnected totality. Heraclitus, with his famous maxim "everything flows" (panta rhei), saw the universe as a constant movement, where all things were in transformation and opposites, far from canceling each other out, actually complemented each other. For him, the harmony of the cosmos resided precisely in this incessant flow, in which unity could only be understood through the interaction between opposites. Change was not a disruption of order, but the very essence of existence.

On the other hand, Parmenides walked in the opposite direction, arguing that being was one, immutable, and indivisible. For him, the multiplicity and change perceived in the world were illusory, the result of a mistaken perception of the senses. True knowledge should be based on reason, which would reveal reality as a cohesive and static whole. The apparent divergence between Heraclitus and Parmenides, far from invalidating their contributions, demonstrated the richness of Greek philosophical thought by exploring the duality between permanence and transformation, unity and multiplicity, anticipating debates that would span the centuries.

Plato, influenced by this tradition, refined the notion of totality in his theory of forms. For him, the sensible world, as we perceive it, was only an imperfect shadow of a higher and immutable reality. The ideal forms – absolute concepts like justice, beauty, and truth – existed fully and perfectly on a transcendent plane, while everything we experience in concrete reality was an imperfect manifestation of these essences. Thus, for Plato, understanding the whole meant going beyond appearances and accessing the underlying structure of reality, where everything was integrated into a larger unity.

His disciple, Aristotle, although he had a more empirical approach and focused on the observation of the natural world, also maintained the importance of understanding phenomena within a larger context. In his metaphysics, he introduced the concept of "final cause" (telos), stating that each being has an inherent purpose that links it to the whole. For Aristotle, the full understanding of any entity could only be achieved by considering its function and its role within the grand scheme of the universe. His thinking paved the way for approaches that reconciled the study of the parts without losing sight of the totality of existence.

In the modern period, holism continued to develop, although often in contrast with the growing reductionism of emerging science. Baruch Spinoza proposed a radically unitary view of reality in his work Ethics, where he argued that God and nature were a single infinite substance (Deus sive Natura). For him, everything in the universe was an expression of this unique substance, and the apparent distinctions between beings were merely different modes of this same fundamental reality. This pantheistic perspective not only reinforced the idea of interconnection between all things but also served as a basis for more integrative conceptions of existence.

Gottfried Wilhelm Leibniz, in turn, formulated the theory of "monads," indivisible entities that composed all reality. Although each monad was autonomous, all were harmonized in a "pre-established harmony," that is, a divinely orchestrated arrangement that ensured the coherence of the universe. This conception emphasized the interdependence between all parts of the cosmos, suggesting that, even though each element seemed to act in isolation, in reality, it participated in a cohesive and well-structured whole.

With the arrival of the 20th century, the notion of holism expanded beyond philosophy, influencing fields such as biology, physics, and systems theory. Alfred North Whitehead, in Process and Reality, formulated a philosophy of process, in which he argued that reality should not be seen as a collection of static objects, but as a continuous flow of interconnected events. For him, each event was shaped by its relationships with other events, emphasizing the importance of interdependence and dynamism in the structure of the cosmos.

Ken Wilber, one of the most influential contemporary thinkers in the field of holism, developed an integral approach that seeks to unify science, philosophy, and spirituality. In his theory of the "spectrum of consciousness," he argues that reality can be understood in multiple layers, from the most material aspects to the most subtle and spiritual ones. For Wilber, a truly holistic vision must integrate different perspectives and levels of analysis, recognizing that each level of existence is intrinsically linked to the others.

In addition to its theoretical implications, holism also carries important ethical repercussions. If everything in the universe is interconnected, then our actions not only affect ourselves but also reverberate throughout the web of existence. This perspective invites us to act with responsibility, empathy, and awareness of the consequences of our actions. Martin Buber, in I and Thou, emphasized the importance of authentic and dialogical relationships, in which we see the other not as an object to be used (It), but as a genuine being worthy of recognition (Thou). This mode of relationship reinforces the holistic principle that existence can only be fully understood in the interconnection between individuals.

Thus, holism, from its beginnings in Greek philosophy to its contemporary formulation, has been an essential pillar for the development of human thought. It teaches us that reality cannot be fragmented into isolated parts, because its true essence lies in the connections that unite all things. By adopting this vision, we can achieve a deeper understanding of existence and act in a more harmonious way in the world.

This broader understanding of reality also challenges us to rethink the way we structure knowledge and organize our societies. Western thought, for a long time, privileged specialization and fragmentation of knowledge, which, despite having driven significant advances in science and technology, often led us to lose sight of the fundamental relationships between phenomena. Today, however, we face an era in which the complexity of global problems requires a more integrated approach. Environmental, social, and technological issues are interconnected, and only a thought that considers these connections can provide effective answers to contemporary challenges.

This need for a more systemic view is reflected in various areas of knowledge, from integrative medicine, which seeks to understand health as a balance between body, mind, and environment, to quantum physics, which demonstrates the interdependence of subatomic particles. In the social sphere, movements that advocate for a circular economy and a sustainable development model also start from this holistic principle, recognizing that human well-being depends on harmony with the environment and with the systems in which we are inserted. This resignification of holism in the 21st century thus represents a return to an ancestral wisdom, now supported by new discoveries and scientific perspectives.

If there is something that the trajectory of holistic thought teaches us, it is that reality cannot be understood without taking into account the connections that structure it. Whether in philosophy, science, or ethics, the idea that the whole and the parts mutually influence each other invites us to see the world with greater depth and responsibility. The future of humanity depends, in large part, on our ability to recognize this interdependence and act from it, promoting a more balanced and conscious coexistence between individuals, societies, and nature.

Chapter 4
Quantum Physics, Biology and Ecology

Contemporary science reveals a deeply interconnected reality, in which natural phenomena cannot be understood in isolation, but as parts of a dynamic and interdependent system. The advancement of knowledge has shown that both the smallest structures of the universe and living and ecological systems function through complex relationships, in which each element influences and is influenced by the whole. This perspective challenges the traditional mechanistic view, which sought to understand nature by breaking it down into smaller parts. Instead, it becomes evident that natural processes operate in an integrated way, suggesting that a full understanding of reality requires a holistic view. This approach has been fundamental to advances in various areas of knowledge, revealing connections that were previously unnoticed and allowing new theories to be formulated based on the interdependence of phenomena.

In physics, biology and ecology, holistic thinking has played a central role in highlighting that the interaction between the components of a system generates emergent properties that cannot be predicted by the isolated analysis of its parts. On a subatomic scale, quantum phenomena demonstrate that seemingly separate particles can be correlated instantaneously, regardless of the distance that separates them, challenging classical conceptions of space and time. In the study of living organisms, it is observed that their functions depend on an intricate network of cellular and biochemical interactions, making it impossible to understand life without taking into account the totality of its processes. In ecology, it is realized that the survival of any species is directly linked to the balance of the environment in which it lives, showing that nature operates as a unified and dynamic system.

This integrated view not only broadens scientific understanding, but also transforms the way human beings interact with the world. The awareness that every action impacts the whole leads us to rethink models of development, production and coexistence, promoting more sustainable and ethical approaches to deal with the challenges of the 21st century. Interdisciplinarity emerges as an essential element for the solution of global problems, uniting knowledge from different fields to deal with issues such as climate change, environmental degradation and collective health. Thus, holism in science not only provides a framework for understanding the complexity of the universe, but also guides practices and decisions that aim at the harmony between natural and human systems, driving a more integrated and responsible vision of reality.

Quantum physics has brought about a revolution in the way we understand reality by revealing that the universe operates in a deeply interconnected way. One of the most fascinating phenomena in this field is quantum entanglement, in which two particles can become so intimately linked that the change in the state of one influences the other instantaneously, regardless of the distance that separates them. This characteristic challenges the classical view of a fragmented world and suggests an underlying unity that transcends traditional notions of space and time. Albert Einstein, intrigued by this peculiarity, referred to it as "spooky action at a distance," recognizing the complexity of the phenomenon, even without fully accepting it.

In addition to entanglement, another fundamental principle of quantum physics is that of uncertainty, formulated by Werner Heisenberg. He established that it is not possible to simultaneously measure with accuracy the position and momentum of a particle. This limitation does not stem from instrumental failures, but from the very nature of the universe, which behaves in a probabilistic and interdependent way. This implies that the observer and the observed phenomenon are not dissociated; on the contrary, the presence of the observer directly influences the outcome of the measurement. With this, quantum physics challenges the conception of a universe composed of isolated entities, revealing that everything is part of a dynamic network of interactions.

If on a subatomic scale the interconnection is a fundamental principle, in biology, holism manifests itself in the organization of living beings. The Systems Theory, proposed by Ludwig von Bertalanffy, argues that organisms cannot be reduced to mere collections of independent parts, as they function as open systems in constant interaction with the environment. Each cell, tissue and organ contributes to the balance of the whole, operating in a harmony that transcends the sum of the individual parts.

A notable example of this perspective is the concept of emergence, in which new and complex characteristics arise from the interaction between simpler components. Human consciousness well illustrates this idea: it cannot be explained only by the isolated analysis of neurons, as it emerges from the complex network of connections between them. In the same way, properties such as the self-organization and adaptation of organisms demonstrate that life is structured in a holistic way, with each element playing a fundamental role for the functioning of the system as a whole.

In addition, biology also shows the interdependence of living beings through symbiotic relationships. Many species coexist in associations that guarantee mutual benefits, as happens between the roots of plants and mycorrhizal fungi. This interaction allows plants to absorb nutrients from the soil more efficiently, while fungi obtain carbohydrates essential for their survival. This type of cooperation is not an exception, but rather a rule in nature, showing that life is sustained through a network of interrelations.

In ecology, the holistic perspective becomes even more evident when considering ecosystems as highly interconnected systems. James Lovelock, through the Gaia Theory, suggested that the Earth behaves as a self-regulating living organism, in which biosphere, atmosphere, oceans and soil interact to maintain conditions favorable to life. This model suggests that the elements of the planet do not operate in isolation, but are connected by natural cycles that guarantee stability and balance to the environment.

A classic example of the holistic functioning of ecology are food chains and webs, in which each organism occupies an essential role. Primary producers, such as plants, sustain herbivores, which in turn serve as food for predators. The removal of a single species can trigger cascade effects, destabilizing the entire ecosystem. This phenomenon highlights the need to preserve biodiversity, as the extinction of a species can compromise the survival of countless others that depend on it directly or indirectly.

Another crucial aspect of ecology is the resilience of ecosystems, which corresponds to the ability to recover from disturbances, such as natural disasters or human actions. Healthy ecological systems, characterized by a rich diversity of organisms and interactions, tend to be more resilient, as they possess natural mechanisms of compensation and adaptation. This understanding reinforces the importance of sustainable practices and environmental conservation, as a degraded ecosystem loses its capacity for regeneration and can collapse.

In view of these findings, modern science has increasingly recognized the need for a holistic approach to understand and solve the challenges of the contemporary world. The science of complex systems, for example, investigates how patterns and properties emerge from the interaction of multiple components, applying this knowledge to diverse areas, from meteorology to economics. Interdisciplinarity, therefore, becomes an essential tool to deal with global problems, such as climate change and the loss of biodiversity.

By adopting an integrated view, we realize that it is not possible to treat environmental, social and scientific issues in an isolated way. Effective solutions require the consideration of the interrelationships between different areas of knowledge, promoting strategies that encompass the multiple aspects of reality. Thus, holism in science not only broadens our understanding of the universe, but also guides decisions that seek greater balance between humanity and nature, ensuring a more sustainable and harmonious future.

This new scientific perspective invites us to deeply rethink the relationship between human beings and the natural world. If everything is interconnected, then our actions, however small they may seem, reverberate on scales much larger than we imagine. Environmental degradation, for example, does not only affect distant ecosystems, but returns in the form of climate change, water crises and collapses in biodiversity that directly impact our quality of life. Similarly, advances in medicine and biotechnology show that caring for human health requires considering not only isolated biological aspects, but also environmental, social and psychological factors, recognizing that individual well-being is inserted in a broader context.

This integrated vision gains even more relevance when applied to economic and social models. Production systems based on the unbridled exploitation of natural resources prove unsustainable in the long term, leading to the search for alternatives such as the regenerative economy and agroecology, which respect the cycles of nature and promote balance between development and conservation. Similarly, effective public policies must take into account the interconnection between environmental, educational and health factors, ensuring fairer and more comprehensive solutions to the challenges of contemporary society. The recognition that each element influences the whole reinforces the importance of collaborative and transdisciplinary approaches in building a more sustainable future.

By unifying knowledge from physics, biology and ecology under a holistic view, we realize that science not only describes reality, but also guides us on how to interact with it in a more harmonious way. The understanding that we live in an interconnected universe invites us to adopt a more responsible role in our daily choices, whether in conscious consumption, in the preservation of the environment or in the valorization of more empathetic and cooperative human relations. If we want to guarantee a viable future for the next generations, we must recognize that the separation between nature and humanity is just an illusion – and that the balance of the whole depends on the consciousness and actions of each part.

Chapter 5
The Quest for Unity

Spirituality has always been rooted in the search for understanding the essential unity that permeates all existence. Since ancient times, various spiritual traditions have developed concepts that emphasize the interconnection between human beings, the universe, and the divine or transcendent principle. This holistic view not only recognizes the presence of an underlying order to reality but also proposes that the separation between beings is, to a large extent, an illusion generated by limited perception. Throughout history, spirituality has served as a means of dissolving this illusion, promoting the idea that each individual is an expression of a larger whole, interconnected by visible and invisible forces that sustain life. Thus, whether through contemplation, meditation, or ritual practices, spiritual experience seeks to transcend fragmentation and reveal the inherent harmony of existence.

Examining different spiritual traditions reveals a common denominator in the valuation of the fundamental unity of the universe. In the East, systems like Hinduism and Buddhism teach that true reality transcends the apparent distinctions between beings and that spiritual awakening occurs when this essential interdependence is perceived. In the West, mystical currents within Christianity and Islam also describe states of deep communion with the divine, in which the separation between self and other dissolves. Beyond these great traditions, spiritual systems more closely tied to nature, such as indigenous beliefs and Shintoism, reflect a holistic understanding of the world, in which every element of creation is seen as sacred and part of a living, dynamic whole. In this way, spirituality, regardless of its cultural origin, invites the individual to perceive themselves not as an isolated entity, but as a link in a vast network of cosmic relations.

In the contemporary world, this holistic vision of spirituality reemerges as a response to the existential and environmental crises that mark the modern era. Faced with the fragmentation promoted by materialism and individualism, the need for an approach that rescues the sense of belonging to a larger whole grows. Contemporary spirituality often integrates ancestral wisdom with scientific discoveries, proposing that consciousness, matter, and energy form an inseparable web. Movements such as spiritual ecology and contemplative practices gain strength by offering paths to restore the connection between human beings and the planet, recognizing that individual healing is directly linked to the balance of the world around them. In this way, holistic spirituality not only broadens the understanding of reality, but also inspires a more harmonious and conscious way of life, guided by the recognition of the interdependence that unites all forms of existence.

Unity in Spiritual Traditions manifests in various forms throughout the religious and philosophical traditions of the world, reflecting a common perception that ultimate reality is an indivisible totality. In Hinduism, this principle is represented by the concept of Brahman, the absolute and transcendent essence that permeates all things. Described as the supreme reality, Brahman is beyond the distinctions and dualities of common existence. According to the Vedic scriptures and the Upanishads, achieving the perception of this unity is the ultimate goal of the spiritual journey. Hindu sages teach that individual identity, or atman, is not separate from Brahman, but rather a manifestation of it. The realization of this principle, known as moksha, occurs when the illusion of separation dissolves, allowing the individual to understand their true nature as an inseparable part of the whole.

In Buddhism, the fundamental interconnectedness of existence is expressed by the concept of pratītyasamutpāda, or dependent origination. This view suggests that everything that exists arises in relation to other things, without a fixed or independent essence. The central teaching of Buddha emphasizes that the idea of a separate self is illusory, a mental construct that generates suffering. Liberation, or nirvana, occurs when this illusion is transcended and the absolute interdependence between all phenomena is perceived. Buddhist spiritual practice, including meditation and mindfulness, aims to dissolve the mistaken perception of separation, allowing the practitioner to experience the unity inherent in reality.

In Taoism, this idea of unity is manifested in the conception of the Tao, the universal force that flows through all things and that transcends intellectual understanding. The Tao Te Ching, a fundamental work attributed to Laozi, describes the Tao as the fundamental principle of existence, a natural flow that should be followed rather than resisted. Spiritual practice in Taoism consists of aligning oneself with this flow, recognizing that all dualities – light and shadow, yin and yang, life and death – are expressions of a single underlying reality. For the Taoist practitioner, harmony arises when this interdependence is accepted and one lives in accordance with the natural rhythm of the universe, rather than trying to impose artificial control over life.

The Experience of Unity is described in various spiritual traditions as a mystical state in which the perception of separation disappears, giving way to a profound sense of belonging to the whole. In Christianity, this experience is reported by mystics such as St. John of the Cross and St. Teresa of Ávila, who described moments of fusion with the divine in which the individual self dissolves in the presence of God. St. John of the Cross, in his poem "Dark Night of the Soul," speaks of a spiritual journey in which the individual's identity is absorbed by divine light, resulting in an experience of absolute love and unity. For St. Teresa, this state of union manifests as a deep ecstasy, in which the soul perceives itself immersed in God, without distinction between subject and object.

In Sufism, the mystical tradition of Islam, the search for unity with God is expressed through the concept of fana, which means the annihilation of the ego in the divine presence. Sufis see this dissolution of the self as the goal of the spiritual journey, a process in which the individual transcends the limitations of personal identity and experiences the totality of Being. The Sufi poet Rumi captured this experience in his verses, describing divine love as a fire that consumes individuality, leaving only the essential truth of existence. For Rumi, God is not separate from the world, but present in all things, and true spiritual realization occurs when this inherent unity is recognized.

Spirituality and Nature also play a fundamental role in understanding cosmic unity. In many indigenous traditions, the Earth is revered as a sacred mother, and all living beings are considered part of a great interconnected web. Among the native peoples of North America, for example, spirituality is deeply rooted in the relationship with nature, where mountains, rivers, and animals are seen as endowed with spirit and consciousness. Respect for nature is not just an ecological issue, but an essential spiritual principle that sustains harmony between humans and the world around them.

In Shintoism, the traditional religion of Japan, the sanctity of nature is expressed in the concept of kami, spirits that inhabit mountains, forests, rivers, and even inanimate objects. Shinto rituals seek to honor these spirits, recognizing that human life is deeply connected to the natural environment. The preservation of nature is not seen merely as a material necessity, but as a sacred duty, for destroying nature is considered an act of disrespect to the kami. This vision inspires practices that emphasize balance and reverence for the natural world, promoting a way of life in tune with the rhythms of the universe.

In the modern world, the need to reconnect with this holistic vision of existence has led many people to seek forms of spirituality that integrate ancient wisdom with contemporary discoveries. Spirituality in the Modern World manifests in movements such as spiritual ecology, which combines environmental concern with a spiritual understanding of nature. This approach recognizes that the environmental crisis is, in its essence, also a spiritual crisis – a reflection of the disconnection between humanity and the planet. Many spiritual traditions teach that caring for the Earth is not just an ecological responsibility, but a sacred act, and that restoring this connection can be a path to healing both the individual and the world around them.

Meditation and other contemplative practices have gained prominence as tools for cultivating this awareness of unity. Techniques such as mindfulness, transcendental meditation, and yoga help to calm the mind and expand perception, allowing the practitioner to experience a deep sense of interconnection with everything around them. These practices not only provide psychological well-being, but also promote a change in the way individuals relate to the world, encouraging a more compassionate, sustainable, and aligned lifestyle with the principles of unity and harmony.

In this way, contemporary spirituality does not only seek metaphysical answers, but also solutions to the concrete challenges of existence. By recognizing that the healing of the planet and spiritual realization are interlinked, a new paradigm emerges that values the interdependence between all beings. Whether through ancient traditions or new interpretations of spirituality, the search for unity continues to be a central axis of the human journey, inspiring more conscious and harmonious ways of living.

This search for unity, present in the most diverse spiritual traditions, reflects a deep longing of the human being for belonging and meaning. In an increasingly fragmented world, where individuality is often exalted at the expense of collectivity, the rescue of this integrated vision becomes essential. The understanding that the separation between beings is an illusion not only transforms the way we see ourselves, but also directly influences our interpersonal relationships and our connection with the planet. When we realize that we are part of a larger whole, we begin to act with more empathy, responsibility, and respect, recognizing that every gesture, however small, reverberates in the great web of existence.

However, this journey towards unity is not limited to the realm of traditional spirituality. In many respects, contemporary science has corroborated this vision, demonstrating that interdependence is a fundamental characteristic of reality. Quantum physics suggests that the separation between matter and energy is illusory, while ecology shows that the survival of each being depends on the balance of the ecosystem around it. This dialogue between spirituality and science strengthens the idea that unity is not just a philosophical or religious concept, but a fundamental truth of existence. Thus, the reunion with this perspective can be the key to facing the challenges of the present, promoting a more harmonious and sustainable way of life.

Throughout history, the search for unity has guided humanity along diverse paths, whether in the silent contemplation of monks, in the ritual dances of ancestral peoples, or in the research of scientists trying to decipher the mysteries of the cosmos. In the end, all these approaches converge on the same perception: we are all parts of a greater whole, interconnected in ways that we often do not fully understand. And perhaps the greatest lesson of this journey is precisely this—there is no separation between us and the universe, between the spiritual and the material, between the past and the future. There is only the continuous flow of existence, inviting us, at every moment, to awaken to the profound unity that connects us.

Chapter 6
The Gaia Hypothesis

The notion that the Earth operates as a living, dynamic system gains scientific support from the Gaia Hypothesis, proposed by James Lovelock. This theory presents Earth as an integrated system where living organisms and physical components interact continuously to maintain conditions conducive to life. Unlike traditional views that analyze the planet's elements in isolation, the Gaia Hypothesis highlights the interdependence between the biosphere, atmosphere, hydrosphere, and geosphere, arguing that life itself actively influences the environment's stability. This perspective suggests that biological processes are not merely products of the terrestrial environment but play an essential role in its regulation, creating a dynamic balance over time. The concept of Gaia not only broadens our understanding of how the planet works but also challenges conventional approaches to science, proposing a systemic model in which interactions between organisms and their environment determine Earth's habitability.

The central idea of the hypothesis does not imply that Earth has consciousness or intention but rather that its natural processes operate in a self-regulating manner, much like a living organism maintains its homeostasis. Evidence suggests that the composition of the atmosphere, for example, is not a passive reflection of chemical and physical processes but a result of the interaction between life and the environment. The stability of oxygen levels, climate regulation, and the maintenance of ocean salinity are some of the mechanisms that support this view. The balance of atmospheric gases, such as oxygen and carbon dioxide, occurs because photosynthetic organisms adjust the air composition, while chemical reactions and geological processes complement this regulation. This systemic model demonstrates how life, from microorganisms to complex ecosystems, shapes and is shaped by the environment in a continuous cycle of adjustments and responses. Lovelock's proposal, therefore, establishes a new paradigm for studying the planet, encouraging a more integrated and holistic approach to ecological and geophysical relationships.

The Gaia Hypothesis also raises questions about the impact of human activity on the planet's balance. If life, over billions of years, has actively participated in maintaining ideal conditions for its own existence, the rapid environmental modification caused by humans may represent a threat to this stability. Climate change, pollution, and the destruction of ecosystems disrupt natural regulation mechanisms, altering Earth's ability to adapt and maintain balance. This view reinforces the need for broader and more sustainable thinking, in which humanity recognizes its participation in the terrestrial system as a whole. Understanding Earth from

Gaia's perspective leads us to consider that any intervention in the environment should be analyzed not only in its immediate effects but in its influence on the global processes that sustain life.

The origin of the Gaia Hypothesis dates back to the 1970s when scientist James Lovelock, in collaboration with microbiologist Lynn Margulis, was developing methods to detect life on other planets in service of NASA. During his research, Lovelock began to realize that the Earth's atmosphere was not just a passive reflection of physical and chemical processes but the result of a constant interaction between living organisms and their environment. This insight led to the formulation of the hypothesis that Earth, as a whole, functions as a dynamic and self-regulating system, capable of maintaining conditions conducive to life over time.

The name "Gaia" was suggested by writer William Golding, a friend of Lovelock, inspired by the Greek goddess who personifies the Earth. The choice of this name reinforced the idea of a living planet in which biological and geological processes work together to ensure its stability. Lovelock adopted this term to emphasize the interdependence between natural elements and life, challenging the fragmented view that predominated in science until then. His proposal did not imply that Earth had consciousness or intention but that its natural mechanisms operated similarly to the homeostasis of a living organism.

The Gaia Hypothesis is based on some fundamental principles that describe how the planet's components interact to maintain the balance necessary for life. One of the central aspects of this hypothesis is the concept of feedback, which regulates essential factors such as temperature, atmospheric composition, and ocean salinity. A classic example is climate regulation. The concentration of gases in the atmosphere, such as carbon dioxide (CO_2) and methane (CH_4), has a direct influence on global temperature. When there is an increase in temperature, certain biological processes, such as photosynthesis, can intensify, absorbing more CO_2 and reducing the greenhouse effect. This negative feedback mechanism helps to avoid extreme temperature variations, maintaining habitable conditions.

Another significant example of terrestrial self-regulation is maintaining ocean salinity. Rivers constantly transport mineral salts to the seas, which could, over time, increase salinity to levels incompatible with life. However, this excessive accumulation does not occur due to the action of biological and geological processes, such as the formation of sediments and the action of marine microorganisms that remove salts from the water. This dynamic balance prevents oceans from becoming excessively salty and ensures the survival of aquatic ecosystems.

The conception of Earth as a living system emphasizes the interconnection between its components and the importance of understanding it in an integrated way. The Gaia Hypothesis invites us to abandon the fragmented view of the planet and recognize that all forms of life, from microorganisms to the most complex ecosystems, play fundamental roles in maintaining environmental conditions. This systemic perspective aligns with modern Earth system science, which studies the interaction between the planet's biotic and abiotic elements.

Although the Gaia Hypothesis was received with skepticism in its early years, its fundamental ideas have been incorporated into contemporary scientific thinking. Initially, many scientists questioned the hypothesis, arguing that it lacked concrete evidence and that the idea of a self-regulating planet seemed exaggerated. However, with the advancement of research on biogeochemical cycles, it became clear that living organisms play an essential role in regulating the terrestrial environment. Studies have shown that the composition of the atmosphere, global temperature, and other environmental factors are not mere products of chance but reflect complex interactions between the biosphere and the other components of the planet.

Currently, the Gaia Hypothesis is widely recognized as a valuable contribution to Earth system science. Although the idea that Earth functions as a living organism still generates debate, the concept that it operates as an interdependent system is widely accepted. The understanding that life actively influences the environment has helped to reshape how we study climate change, ecology, and geophysics.

The implications of this hypothesis go beyond science and directly touch on environmental issues and humanity's relationship with the planet. If Earth has been able to maintain favorable conditions for life for billions of years, human actions may represent a significant threat to this balance. Pollution, deforestation, and the excessive emission of greenhouse gases disrupt natural regulation mechanisms and can compromise the planet's climatic and ecological stability. Global warming, increased ocean acidity, and biodiversity loss are examples of how human activities affect the natural processes that sustain life.

The perspective offered by the Gaia Hypothesis leads us to reflect on the need for a more holistic and sustainable approach to dealing with environmental challenges. Instead of treating problems such as global warming or species extinction in isolation, we must consider the connections between all elements of the terrestrial system. Solutions to environmental crises cannot be limited to palliative measures; it is necessary to adopt integrated strategies that take into account the interdependence between climate, biodiversity, water resources, and human activities.

In this way, the Gaia Hypothesis teaches us that every action has repercussions throughout the planetary system. If we want to guarantee a sustainable future, it is essential to recognize our active participation in the terrestrial dynamics and assume responsibility for preserving the balance that has allowed the existence of life for so long. This vision not only transforms our scientific understanding of the Earth but also reinforces the need for a collective commitment to preserving the environment.

Over the decades, the Gaia Hypothesis has inspired new scientific and philosophical approaches to the relationship between life and the environment. Its impact goes beyond academia, influencing ecological movements, environmental policies, and even environmental ethics. The idea that Earth functions as a self-regulating system reinforces the urgency of rethinking our role on the planet, not as dominators of nature, but as active participants in a balance that has been built for billions of years. This change of perspective suggests that, instead of exploiting natural resources without considering their consequences, we should learn from the natural mechanisms of regulation and adaptation that Earth itself offers us.

By integrating this systemic vision into our understanding of the planet, we can develop technologies and strategies that work in harmony with natural processes, minimizing negative impacts and promoting a sustainable development model. Earth system science, driven by ideas derived from the Gaia Hypothesis, continues to advance, revealing how interactions between organisms and the environment shape the future of life on the planet. The growing awareness of climate change and the need for energy transitions are reflections of this broader understanding, which leads us to consider solutions based on natural cycles and regenerative processes.

Thus, the Gaia Hypothesis remains a reminder that Earth is not just a stage for life but a living system in itself, in which each element plays a fundamental role in maintaining environmental conditions. Recognizing this interdependence challenges us to act with more responsibility and sensitivity in the face of the ecological crises we face. True sustainability will only be achieved when we see Earth not as a resource to be exploited but as an organism of which we are a part, whose health and balance are essential for the continuity of life.

Chapter 7
Respecting the Interconnectedness of Life

The understanding of the interconnectedness between all life forms on the planet transforms the way human beings perceive their role in the natural world. Deep ecology emerges as a response to the reductionist and utilitarian view that has historically dominated relations between humanity and the environment. Instead of considering nature merely as a resource to be exploited, this approach proposes a radical transformation in the way people interact with ecosystems, recognizing the intrinsic interdependence between all living beings. This perspective is not limited to technical adjustments or palliative solutions to environmental problems, but seeks a revolution in human consciousness, culture and values, promoting an integrated and respectful view of life. By stating that each being has an intrinsic value, regardless of its usefulness to humanity, deep ecology challenges the dominant mentality and invites society to reassess its attitudes, policies and habits in relation to the planet.

This new philosophical and environmental approach emphasizes that the ecological crisis is not just a technical problem to be solved with scientific innovations, but a crisis of values that requires profound changes in the way we think and act. The degradation of ecosystems, the loss of biodiversity and the climate collapse are not isolated events, but symptoms of a misguided paradigm that separates humans from nature and places them in a position of dominance. Deep ecology proposes, in contrast, a model of coexistence in which humanity recognizes its insertion in a complex web of life, where all species play essential roles in the balance of the planet. This vision challenges the traditional hierarchical structure that places human interests above other living beings and suggests a shift to a biocentric model, where every organism has the right to exist and flourish within its own ecological context.

By adopting this perspective, deep ecology inspires practices and movements aimed at building a sustainable and regenerative future. The valorization of biological and cultural diversity, the search for simpler and more sustainable lifestyles, and the defense of ecological justice are some of the principles that emerge from this philosophy. Self-sustaining communities, permaculture, restoration of degraded ecosystems and ecological education are practical examples of how this vision can be applied in everyday life. Although it is the target of criticism for its radicalism and for questioning consolidated socioeconomic structures, deep ecology presents a way to rethink the relationship between humanity and nature, promoting a more balanced and harmonious world. This transformation does not occur only through political or economic changes, but through a collective awakening to the interconnectivity of life and the shared responsibility to preserve the planet for future generations.

The term "deep ecology" was coined by the Norwegian philosopher Arne Naess in 1973, marking an essential distinction between a superficial approach to ecology and a more philosophical and holistic understanding of the relationship between humanity and nature. For Naess, the environmental crisis transcends the technical sphere and is rooted in a problem of values and worldview. While traditional ecology often focuses on solving environmental problems through pragmatic and palliative measures, deep ecology proposes a more comprehensive revolution in the way human beings perceive their connection with the planet.

The basis of this philosophy was strongly influenced by various spiritual and philosophical traditions, such as Buddhism and Taoism, which emphasize harmony with nature, in addition to indigenous worldviews that have always sustained a relationship of respect and reciprocity with the environment. Holistic thinking has also contributed significantly, providing a systemic perspective on natural processes and the interdependence between organisms. In addition, figures such as Rachel Carson, author of Silent Spring, and Aldo Leopold, with his land ethic expressed in A Sand County Almanac, offered fundamental contributions by highlighting the impacts of human action on ecosystems and the need for a more ethical and responsible approach.

In an attempt to structure this vision, Arne Naess and George Sessions elaborated, in 1984, a set of fundamental principles that define deep ecology. The first principle establishes the intrinsic value of all forms of life, regardless of their usefulness to human beings. This concept breaks with the predominant anthropocentric mentality, recognizing that every organism has the right to existence and development within its own ecological niche. Biological and cultural diversity is equally valued, as it ensures the resilience of ecosystems and strengthens the adaptation of living beings to environmental changes.

Another essential principle of deep ecology is the need for change in human behavior. To ensure the health of the planet, it is imperative to reduce excessive interference in ecosystems and adopt simpler and more sustainable lifestyles. This implies a review of consumption patterns, greater awareness of the environmental impact of human activities and an effort to align daily practices with ecological balance.

Ecological justice also occupies a central role within this perspective. The indiscriminate exploitation of nature is directly linked to the marginalization of vulnerable communities, especially those that depend directly on natural resources for their survival. In this way, the struggle for environmental preservation cannot be dissociated from the search for social equity, as both aspects are deeply intertwined.

The interdependence between all living beings reinforces this vision, as it shows that human well-being is intrinsically connected to the health of the planet. When ecosystems are destroyed or altered irreversibly, the impacts fall not only on the species that inhabit them, but also on the human populations that depend on ecosystem services for their survival, such as clean water, clean air and fertile soil.

Deep ecology also proposes an expanded notion of self-realization, encouraging individuals to perceive themselves as part of a living and interconnected web, instead of isolated agents in a fragmented world. This understanding transforms the way people see their identity and purpose, fostering a feeling of belonging and responsibility towards the environment.

In the political and social sphere, the decentralization of power is pointed out as a viable way to promote greater sustainability. Self-sustaining local communities, based on cooperative and participatory models, can play a crucial role in building fairer and more resilient societies. This implies a redistribution of decisions to levels closer to local realities, allowing for more efficient and respectful management of natural resources.

In addition, deep ecology defends direct and non-violent action as a legitimate means of promoting ecological justice and protecting the environment. Demonstrations, boycotts and practices of peaceful resistance become fundamental tools to pressure for changes and raise awareness in society about the urgency of the environmental crisis.

The adoption of a holistic view of nature is one of the central characteristics of deep ecology, as it rejects the notion that humanity occupies a superior place in the hierarchy of life. Instead, it proposes that human beings recognize their role within a larger and interdependent system, in which each organism has an essential function. This shift in perspective has profound implications for consumption patterns, economic models and social relations, encouraging more responsible and harmonious practices.

This approach translates into a series of practical applications that encompass various areas of everyday life. In the agricultural sector, for example, deep ecology promotes sustainable cultivation methods, such as permaculture and organic agriculture, which respect natural cycles and minimize environmental impact. Ecological restoration is another essential aspect, with initiatives aimed at recovering degraded areas and conserving biodiversity.

The encouragement of a simpler and more conscious lifestyle is also part of this philosophy. This does not mean giving up comfort or progress, but rethinking consumption habits, reducing waste and prioritizing more sustainable practices. Environmental education plays a fundamental role in this process, as it is through awareness that a lasting transformation in the collective mentality can be promoted.

Despite its valuable contributions, deep ecology is not without criticism. Some argue that its proposal is utopian and difficult to implement within the current globalized and industrialized context. Others point out that the emphasis on reducing human interference can neglect the needs of populations in developing countries, which often depend on the exploitation of natural resources for their subsistence.

However, its defenders argue that the severity of the environmental crisis demands radical changes in the way humanity interacts with the planet. They argue that palliative measures are not sufficient to deal with the ecological challenges of the 21st century and that only a profound transformation in values and habits can guarantee a sustainable future for future generations.

In this way, deep ecology offers not only a set of philosophical principles, but a call to action, encouraging a new relationship between human beings and the natural world. By recognizing the interconnectivity of life and assuming responsibility for the preservation of ecosystems, society can take a significant step towards a more balanced future, where respect for nature and ecological justice are central values.

The adoption of this perspective requires a continuous commitment to change, both at the individual and collective level. Small daily choices, such as reducing resource consumption, supporting sustainable agricultural practices and valuing biodiversity, add up to political and social actions that challenge predatory models of development. The transition to a society more harmonious with nature does not occur instantaneously, but is strengthened as more people become aware of the need to rethink their relations with the natural world.

More than an abstract philosophy, deep ecology invites the practical experimentation of new forms of coexistence and organization. Projects of environmental regeneration, movements of ecological resistance and networks of community support demonstrate that change is possible and that sustainable alternatives are already under construction. The urgency of environmental crises, far from being an obstacle, can serve as a catalyst for a collective transformation, driven by those who recognize the interdependence of life and wish to act in its favor.

The interconnection between all living beings reminds us that our actions reverberate far beyond the immediate present. By recognizing the intrinsic value of nature and assuming a posture of respect and cooperation, humanity has the opportunity to redefine its role on the planet. The construction of a sustainable future depends not only on technological advances or political changes, but on a revolution in the way we perceive and live our relationship with the natural world.

Chapter 8
Holism and Sustainability

The pursuit of a sustainable future demands a profound shift in how we understand and interact with the world. On a planet where environmental, social, and economic challenges are intrinsically linked, it becomes essential to abandon fragmented views and adopt a holistic approach that recognizes the interdependence between all systems. The climate crisis, the depletion of natural resources, social inequality, and economic instability are not isolated problems, but symptoms of a development model that prioritizes immediate gains at the expense of long-term harmony. To overcome these challenges, it is crucial to integrate knowledge, innovation, and ethical values, promoting a vision that respects the limits of nature, ensures social justice, and drives a sustainable economy.

The holistic approach is based on the principle that no effective solution can be found without considering the impact of each action within the larger whole of the global system. Traditional solutions, often limited to specific adjustments, fail to ignore vital connections between different sectors and aspects of human and environmental life. When public policies or technological advances seek to correct a specific problem without taking into account its effect in other areas, the results can be contradictory. For example, intensive agricultural practices increase food production in the short term, but deplete the soil, contaminate water sources, and contribute to deforestation, creating new environmental and social problems. Similarly, energy solutions that reduce carbon emissions can have negative impacts if they are not planned in an integrated way, such as competition between biofuels and food security. Holism proposes that every decision be made with a broad vision, considering how different factors interact and influence each other over time.

Faced with this reality, holistic sustainability presents itself as an essential way to redefine our relationship with the planet and with ourselves. The transition to this model requires structural changes in the economy, culture, and the way we organize our societies, prioritizing a dynamic balance between environmental preservation, economic development, and social well-being. This means encouraging practices such as the circular economy, which reduces waste and optimizes resources; regenerative agriculture, which maintains soil fertility and protects biodiversity; and sustainable urban planning, which integrates green spaces, efficient transportation, and social inclusion. In addition, education plays a central role in this transformation, promoting a collective awareness focused on integrated and long-term solutions. Only by recognizing that all forms of life and human activities are part of an interconnected system will it be possible to build a truly sustainable future, based on harmony between progress and preservation.

The need for a holistic approach becomes evident when we analyze the limitations of traditional sustainability, which often focuses separately on the environmental, social, and economic aspects. This fragmented model can lead to solutions that, while solving a specific problem, create new challenges in other areas. A clear example of this is the production of biofuels, which aims to reduce carbon emissions, but can result in accelerated deforestation and competition for agricultural land, compromising food security and biodiversity. Thus, it is essential to adopt an integrating look, understanding that each action in one sector reverberates throughout the global system.

Holism invites us to see these pillars as interconnected and interdependent, requiring that any sustainable solution take into account the complex interactions between environmental, social, and economic systems. Instead of isolated interventions, we need strategies that address the challenges in their entirety, promoting mutual benefits and avoiding negative side effects. An example of this is the development of reforestation policies that, in addition to capturing carbon, also regenerate ecosystems, protect water sources, and promote social inclusion through the involvement of local communities in environmental restoration. This systemic approach becomes essential to ensure that responses to global challenges are effective and lasting.

Holistic sustainability is based on essential principles that guide the creation of balanced and integrated solutions. The first of these principles is interconnection, which recognizes that all areas of life are linked and that no action occurs in isolation. This means that changes in land use, industrial production, or energy consumption will have impacts that go beyond their direct sectors, affecting biodiversity, climate, and society as a whole.

Balance is another central principle, as it seeks to harmonize environmental, social, and economic needs, ensuring that one of these dimensions is not prioritized at the expense of the others. Sustainable development models should be designed to allow economic growth without compromising the integrity of ecosystems or increasing social inequalities.

Resilience also stands out as an essential pillar. Sustainable systems need to be able to adapt and recover from disturbances, whether they are economic crises, climate change, or natural disasters. Strategies such as diversification of energy sources, strengthening of local agriculture, and implementation of resilient infrastructures are examples of how holistic sustainability can increase the adaptive capacity of society in the face of future challenges.

Another fundamental aspect is justice, which requires the equitable distribution of the benefits and costs of sustainability. This means that environmental policies cannot harm vulnerable communities, and that decisions about the use of natural resources should take into account both current and future generations. The inclusion of marginalized populations in decision-making processes and the implementation of fair compensation mechanisms are strategies that ensure that sustainable progress is truly democratic.

Finally, the long-term vision is indispensable for a holistic approach, as the choices made today will have lasting impacts. Planning cities, infrastructures, and economic models considering their impact for the next generations is fundamental to avoid palliative solutions that only postpone problems. Investments in environmental education, conservation of natural resources, and sustainable technologies are measures that guarantee a balanced and prosperous future.

In practice, holistic sustainability can be applied in various areas, bringing innovative solutions to urban, agricultural, and industrial challenges. In urban planning, for example, a holistic model is not limited to physical infrastructure, but considers quality of life, social inclusion, and environmental resilience. This involves the creation of green spaces that provide well-being and reduce the temperature of cities, the incentive to sustainable public transport, and the integration of technologies that minimize the consumption of energy and resources.

In agriculture, the holistic approach is manifested in the adoption of regenerative practices that seek to restore soil health, conserve water, and protect biodiversity. Techniques such as agroforestry, which combines agricultural species and native trees to create productive and balanced ecosystems, crop rotation to maintain soil fertility, and the use of organic compounds to reduce dependence on synthetic fertilizers are strategies that promote a sustainable food system.

Another significant example is the circular economy, a model that proposes a radical change in the way we use resources. Unlike the linear model of "extract, produce, and discard," the circular economy is based on the reuse, recycling, and regeneration of materials, reducing waste and maximizing efficiency. Companies that adopt this approach invest in biodegradable packaging, production processes that minimize waste, and reverse logistics systems for the reuse of products.

Education also plays an essential role in this process, as a holistic model of teaching goes beyond the transmission of technical information and encourages sustainable values and attitudes. Education for sustainability should emphasize the interconnection of all forms of life and the collective responsibility in the preservation of the planet. Schools and universities can include practices such as community gardens, projects for the reuse of materials, and environmental engagement initiatives to make learning more practical and meaningful.

However, the transition to a holistic sustainability faces considerable challenges. One of the biggest obstacles is the resistance to change, especially in economic and political systems that prioritize immediate gains at the expense of long-term well-being. Reshaping productive chains, rethinking growth models, and integrating ecological principles into public policies require political will, strategic investments, and a joint effort between governments, companies, and civil society.

In addition, the complexity of global systems makes it difficult to predict and manage all the impacts of sustainable actions. A well-intentioned solution can generate unexpected consequences if it is not analyzed comprehensively. Therefore, scientific research and continuous monitoring are indispensable tools to ensure that the strategies implemented truly promote balance and resilience.

Despite these challenges, there are countless opportunities to move towards a more sustainable model. The growing awareness of environmental and social problems has driven the demand for integrated and innovative solutions. Emerging technologies, such as renewable energy sources, artificial intelligence applied to resource management, and biotechnology for environmental regeneration, offer powerful tools for building a more balanced future.

Global collaboration is also essential. The exchange of knowledge, cooperation between nations, and the creation of sustainable innovation networks are fundamental strategies to address challenges that transcend borders, such as climate change and resource scarcity.

While governments and companies play a central role in this process, individuals also have a significant impact on building a more sustainable world. Small changes in lifestyle, such as reducing excessive consumption, choosing products of sustainable origin, avoiding food waste, and supporting local conservation initiatives, contribute to a transformative collective effect. In addition, the dissemination of knowledge and engagement in environmental causes strengthen the culture of sustainability, promoting a mentality that values balance and shared responsibility.

By adopting a holistic approach, we can address global challenges more effectively and build a truly sustainable future. Holistic sustainability is not just a theoretical concept, but a path that requires commitment, innovation, and collaboration to ensure harmony between progress and preservation.

The adoption of this perspective requires a change in the way societies plan their development, recognizing that every decision has broad and interconnected implications. Instead of fragmented and reactive measures, holistic sustainability proposes proactive and systemic strategies, which consider both the immediate impacts and the long-term effects. This requires a collective effort involving governments, companies, academic institutions, and civil society, promoting policies and practices that encourage environmental regeneration, social equity, and the responsible use of natural resources.

This transformation does not mean giving up progress or economic growth, but redefining its parameters so that they are compatible with the resilience of ecosystems and human well-being. Development models that value cooperation, sustainable innovation, and respect for natural cycles demonstrate that it is possible to thrive without compromising the foundations that sustain life on the planet. By integrating different areas of knowledge and considering the interdependence between ecological, social, and economic systems, the way opens for a future in which the balance between humanity and nature is not just an ideal, but a concrete reality.

The challenge of building this future demands not only technological advancements and institutional changes, but also an ethical and cultural commitment to the preservation of life in all its forms. Holistic sustainability is not just about minimizing negative impacts, but about creating regenerative solutions that strengthen ecosystems and promote justice for all generations. By understanding that we are embedded in a web of interdependent relationships, we can act with greater awareness and responsibility, ensuring that the legacy left for the future is one of harmony, abundance, and respect for the complexity of the natural world.

Chapter 9
The Wisdom of Ecosystems

Nature operates as a large, dynamic, interconnected system, where every organism and element plays a fundamental role in maintaining ecological balance. Unlike linear and fragmented models of human organization, ecosystems function through closed loops, efficiently harnessing and transforming resources. This complex web of interdependencies demonstrates that sustainability is not just an abstract concept, but an intrinsic principle of life itself. The ability of ecosystems to self-regulate, adapt to change, and thrive for long periods without generating waste or collapsing demonstrates a natural intelligence that can serve as an inspiration for rethinking our social, economic, and environmental structures. By understanding and applying the principles of ecology, we can build more resilient, collaborative, and harmonious societies, reducing negative impacts and promoting the regeneration of natural resources.

Ecological resilience is one of the most remarkable aspects of nature. Healthy ecosystems not only maintain balance, but also have recovery mechanisms in the face of external disturbances, such as climate change, fires, or the introduction of new species.

This resilience is the result of biological diversity, the interdependence between organisms, and the efficiency of natural cycles. In contrast, human systems that neglect these principles become fragile, dependent on external inputs, and vulnerable to crises. Agricultural monoculture, for example, exemplifies this vulnerability: by prioritizing only one plant species on vast tracts of land, it reduces biodiversity, depletes the soil, and requires the intensive use of fertilizers and pesticides. Learning from ecosystems means adopting practices that promote diversity and regeneration, ensuring long-term stability and reducing the need for artificial interventions to correct imbalances created by the human model of exploitation.

In addition to resilience, ecosystems teach us that competition and cooperation coexist in harmony. Although natural selection drives evolution through competition between species, collaboration is equally essential for survival. Symbiotic relationships, such as pollination by bees or the association between fungi and plant roots, show that cooperation increases efficiency and strengthens systems. This balance can also be applied to human societies, encouraging a more collaborative approach in economics, politics, and social relations. Models based only on exacerbated competition generate inequality and environmental degradation, while initiatives based on cooperation promote innovation, well-being, and sustainability. By observing and learning from ecosystems, we can build a more balanced future, where human development occurs in harmony with nature, and not at its expense.

The interconnection in ecosystems reveals itself as a fundamental principle that sustains the web of life. Each organism, from microscopic bacteria to the imposing predators at the top of the food chain, plays an indispensable role in maintaining ecological balance. The interaction between plants, herbivores, carnivores, and decomposers forms a continuous cycle, where nothing is lost and everything is transformed. Plants, by performing photosynthesis, convert solar energy into food and release oxygen, essential for the respiration of other living beings. Herbivores feed on plants, transferring this energy to another level of the trophic chain. Predators then control the herbivore population, preventing them from consuming excessive vegetation and causing environmental imbalances. Finally, decomposers, such as fungi and bacteria, break down the organic matter of dead organisms, returning nutrients to the soil and closing the cycle of life.

This intricate system teaches us that all actions have consequences that resonate far beyond what we can immediately perceive. The removal of a single species can generate unpredictable impacts, triggering cascading reactions that destabilize the entire ecosystem. For example, the extinction of a natural predator can lead to the uncontrolled growth of the herbivore population, resulting in the degradation of vegetation and, eventually, the scarcity of resources for other species. Similarly, in the human context, our daily choices—whether in the consumption of goods, food, or the use of natural resources—directly affect the environment and society. Ecological interconnection reflects human interdependence, where individual and collective decisions shape the future of the planet.

Biological diversity is another essential pillar for the resilience of ecosystems. Environments rich in biodiversity have a greater capacity for adaptation and recovery in the face of disturbances, such as fires, droughts, or epidemics. When there is a variety of genetic and species, there will always be organisms capable of resisting environmental changes, ensuring the continuity of life. The disappearance of a species can be compensated by another with similar ecological functions, preserving the balance of the system. For example, tropical forests, full of different types of trees, birds, insects, and mammals, are extremely resilient due to their diversity. In contrast, impoverished ecosystems, such as agricultural monocultures, are vulnerable to pests and diseases, as the absence of diversity prevents the system from regulating itself naturally.

This logic also applies to human societies. Diverse communities, composed of people from different cultures, abilities, and perspectives, tend to be more innovative and adaptable to change. When there is diversity of thought, creative solutions emerge to address complex challenges. Companies that value multidisciplinary teams, for example, tend to be more resilient and competitive in the market. Similarly, societies that promote inclusion and respect for differences strengthen their ability to overcome crises and evolve.

In ecosystems, energy and nutrients circulate cyclically, ensuring long-term sustainability. The water cycle, the carbon cycle, and the nitrogen cycle are examples of natural processes that allow the continuous renewal of the essential elements for life. Water, evaporating from the oceans, forms clouds that generate rain, replenishing rivers and aquifers before returning to the seas. Carbon, fundamental to the constitution of living beings, circulates between the atmosphere, organisms, and sediments, being constantly recycled. These natural processes demonstrate the efficiency of ecological systems in keeping resources available indefinitely.

This principle can be applied in the organization of human activities through the concept of a circular economy. Unlike the traditional linear model of "extract, produce, and discard," the circular economy proposes the reuse and recycling of materials, reducing waste and minimizing environmental impacts. Products can be designed to have a long lifespan, and waste can be transformed into new resources. Technologies such as composting organic waste, capturing and reusing rainwater, and recycling plastics and metals follow this logic inspired by natural cycles, promoting a more intelligent and sustainable use of resources.

Adaptation and evolution are inherent characteristics of ecosystems, which constantly adjust to environmental changes. Evolution occurs through natural selection, where the organisms best adapted to certain conditions survive and reproduce, transmitting their characteristics to future generations. Species develop new strategies to deal with predators, find food, or resist adverse conditions. For example, certain desert plants have evolved to store large amounts of water in their tissues, ensuring their survival in arid climates.

In human society, this capacity for adaptation is equally crucial. In a constantly changing world, with technological advances, climate change, and economic challenges, flexibility and resilience are fundamental. Individuals, companies, and governments that manage to reinvent themselves in the face of adversity have a greater chance of prospering. Continuous learning, innovation, and the ability to reformulate strategies are aspects that guarantee survival and progress in the long term.

In ecosystems, competition and cooperation coexist harmoniously. Competition drives evolution by selecting the fittest individuals, while cooperation allows species to benefit each other. Symbiotic relationships, such as the association between mycorrhizal fungi and plant roots, demonstrate how collaboration strengthens natural systems. The fungi provide essential nutrients to the plants, which, in turn, share carbohydrates with the fungi. This type of partnership improves the efficiency of the ecosystem and increases its resilience.

In the same way, in society, both competition and cooperation are essential for development. Companies that compete for innovation drive technological progress, but strategic partnerships between sectors can generate sustainable solutions to global problems. Economic models based exclusively on extreme competition can generate inequality and environmental degradation, while systems that balance collaboration and competition promote prosperity and social balance.

The practical application of the wisdom of ecosystems can revolutionize various areas, from the design of cities to business management. The concept of regenerative design, for example, seeks not only to minimize environmental impacts, but also to restore and strengthen ecosystems. This includes buildings designed to generate more energy than they consume, urban reforestation initiatives, and the creation of green spaces integrated into cities. The sustainable management of natural resources also benefits from this approach, considering the complex interactions between natural and human systems. Strategies such as agroforestry, which combines agricultural species and native trees to restore soils and promote biodiversity, exemplify this application.

In addition, the circular economy, inspired by ecological cycles, transforms waste into resources and promotes the continuous reuse of materials. Companies that adopt this model reduce costs, minimize environmental impacts, and increase their efficiency. Innovative technologies, such as the production of bioplastics from organic waste and decentralized renewable energy systems, demonstrate how nature can serve as an inspiration for more sustainable development.

The wisdom of ecosystems offers us valuable lessons about interconnection, diversity, cycles, adaptation, and cooperation. By learning from nature, we can create more resilient and balanced societies, ensuring a sustainable future for generations to come. Ecological intelligence teaches us that we are not separate from the environment that surrounds us, but we are an integral part of it, and our survival depends on respect and harmony with natural systems.

Understanding the principles that govern ecosystems invites us to rethink the way we structure our societies and interact with the natural world. By adopting nature-inspired approaches, we can create more resilient and sustainable systems, promoting a balanced coexistence between human progress and environmental preservation. Biomimicry, for example, has shown how observing natural processes can inspire innovative solutions in various areas, from the design of materials to urban and industrial management. Nature has already solved many of the challenges we face today, and learning from its strategies may be the key to a more harmonious future.

In addition, the valorization of ecological and social diversity reveals itself as an essential factor for sustainability and innovation. Just as diverse ecosystems are more resilient to changes and challenges, societies that promote inclusion and cultural plurality are better prepared to deal with crises and find creative solutions to complex problems. This implies rethinking development models, prioritizing regenerative, collaborative, and integrated approaches that respect natural rhythms and ensure quality of life for future generations.

The wisdom of ecosystems reminds us that we are not separate entities from nature, but part of a vast interdependent network. Every action we take reverberates in the global balance, affecting not only our species, but all life forms on the planet. By integrating this knowledge into our daily choices and collective decisions, we can tread a path of greater respect, awareness and regeneration. Building a sustainable future means not only minimizing negative impacts, but acting actively to restore and strengthen natural systems, ensuring that life continues to flourish in its fullness.

Chapter 10
Addressing Global Challenges

The climate crisis stands as one of humanity's most comprehensive and pressing challenges, demanding a fundamental shift in how we interact with the planet. Unlike isolated problems that can be resolved with targeted solutions, climate change involves a complex web of environmental, social, economic, and political factors that influence one another. The rise in global temperatures, the intensification of extreme weather events, and the loss of biodiversity are not merely symptoms of an environmental problem, but reflections of an unsustainable development model that has prioritized immediate economic growth at the expense of the stability of natural systems. To effectively address this crisis, it is essential to adopt a holistic approach, recognizing that every action has repercussions across multiple dimensions and that fragmented solutions will not be sufficient to reverse the damage already caused.

A holistic view of climate change requires that we understand the connections between different sectors and regions of the planet. Deforestation in the Amazon, for example, not only affects local biodiversity, but also influences rainfall patterns in other continents, alters the absorption of carbon from the atmosphere, and affects global food security. Similarly, the dependence on fossil fuels not only contributes to global warming, but also perpetuates socioeconomic inequalities, funding polluting industries and delaying the transition to a sustainable economy. Holism teaches us that all human actions are embedded in an interdependent global system, where decisions made in one location can have lasting impacts on a planetary scale. Thus, any solution to the climate crisis needs to integrate environmental, social, and economic aspects, ensuring that progress in emissions reduction and ecological restoration is accompanied by social justice and sustainable prosperity for all populations.

The response to this challenge requires the implementation of coordinated strategies that combine mitigation and adaptation, promote the restoration of ecosystems, and encourage structural changes in consumption and production patterns. The transition to renewable energy sources, for example, cannot occur without considering its impacts on workers and communities dependent on traditional sectors. Similarly, sustainable agricultural policies should ensure food security without compromising soil regeneration and biodiversity preservation. Collaboration between governments, businesses, scientists, and citizens is essential to develop effective solutions and ensure their application on a global scale. In addition, it is fundamental to promote a change of mentality, encouraging a new relationship between society and the environment based on respect, interdependence, and shared responsibility. Only by adopting this integrated and systemic vision can humanity face climate change efficiently and build a more balanced and sustainable future.

Climate change represents a phenomenon of immense complexity, in which multiple elements interact in a delicate balance. The atmosphere, the oceans, the biosphere, and the cryosphere are deeply interconnected, and any alteration in one of these components has repercussions throughout the system. The increase in concentrations of greenhouse gases, such as carbon dioxide (CO_2) and methane (CH_4), has triggered unprecedented global warming, resulting in the melting of polar ice caps and glaciers, the rise in sea levels, the acidification of marine waters, and the intensification of extreme weather events, such as hurricanes, heat waves, and prolonged droughts.

Understanding this complexity requires a look that goes beyond the isolated analysis of each effect, requiring a holistic approach. This perspective allows us to visualize the interactions between the different components of the climate system and understand how such changes impact not only the environment, but also social and economic dynamics on a global scale. The interdependence between natural and human systems highlights the need for integrated solutions, which take into account both the mitigation of the damage already caused and the adaptation to the transformations that will inevitably occur.

Holism offers us an essential key to interpreting climate change as a systemic problem, in which causes and effects are interconnected and feed each other. A clear example of this is the deforestation of the Amazon, which not only intensifies CO_2 emissions by releasing large amounts of carbon stored in trees, but also alters rainfall patterns in distant regions, negatively influencing agriculture and ecosystems of other continents. The loss of this forest compromises water regulation, reducing the humidity transported to other areas and, consequently, affecting agricultural productivity and increasing vulnerability to severe droughts.

Furthermore, holism leads us to reflect on the very root of the climate crisis, which cannot be reduced to a technical or scientific problem. It is also a crisis of values, a direct consequence of the anthropocentric view that for centuries has placed human beings as the center of the universe, treating nature as an inexhaustible resource to be exploited. This reductionist mentality ignores the interdependence between living beings and ecosystems, perpetuating an economic and social model that neglects the limits of the planet. Thus, a truly holistic approach not only proposes technological solutions to reduce emissions or restore ecosystems, but also demands a profound change in the way we conceive our relationship with the natural world.

Given this scenario, addressing climate change effectively requires solutions that integrate multiple aspects, addressing both the causes and the impacts of this phenomenon in a coordinated manner. Among the fundamental strategies for this approach are:

Mitigation and adaptation are complementary and indispensable strategies in the fight against climate change. While mitigation focuses on reducing greenhouse gas emissions, through the transition to clean energy sources, the protection of natural ecosystems, and the adoption of sustainable practices in agriculture and industry, adaptation seeks to prepare communities and infrastructures for the inevitable impacts of the changes already underway. This includes measures such as building barriers against rising sea levels, developing agricultural crops more resistant to droughts and floods, and creating public policies that protect vulnerable populations from climate disasters.

Energy transition is one of the fundamental pillars of mitigation. The replacement of fossil fuels with renewable sources, such as solar, wind, and hydroelectric, is essential to drastically reduce carbon emissions. However, this change must occur in a fair and inclusive way, ensuring that workers in traditional sectors, such as coal and oil, have opportunities for professional retraining and can integrate into the new green economy. In addition, it is necessary to consider the decentralization of energy generation, promoting the use of solar panels in homes and small communities, reducing dependence on large corporations and democratizing access to clean electricity.

Ecosystem restoration is another essential strategy to mitigate the effects of climate change. Tropical forests, mangroves, and wetlands play a crucial role in capturing and storing carbon, helping to regulate the global climate. In addition, healthy ecosystems provide a range of fundamental environmental services, such as water purification, maintenance of biodiversity, and protection against extreme weather events. Reforestation and recovery projects of degraded areas should be encouraged and funded, ensuring that these initiatives involve local communities and respect traditional knowledge about sustainable land management.

Sustainable agriculture emerges as one of the most promising ways to reduce emissions associated with food production and, at the same time, increase the resilience of agricultural systems. Practices such as agroforestry, which combines trees and agricultural crops in the same space, allow for soil regeneration and the absorption of carbon from the atmosphere. Organic agriculture, which dispenses with synthetic fertilizers and pesticides, contributes to the health of ecosystems and food security. In addition, techniques of crop rotation and no-till planting help maintain soil fertility and reduce erosion, ensuring sustainable production in the long term.

Education and awareness play a central role in building a more sustainable society. Informative campaigns and educational programs can help disseminate knowledge about the impacts of climate change and encourage responsible attitudes towards consumption and the environment. Schools and universities have a crucial role in this process, preparing new generations to deal with environmental challenges and foster innovative solutions. At the same time, the media and social networks can be powerful tools to mobilize public opinion and pressure governments and companies to adopt more sustainable policies.

Global collaboration is indispensable to face a challenge of planetary scale. No country can solve the climate crisis alone, and international cooperation is essential to implement effective policies and ensure that the most vulnerable nations receive the necessary support to deal with environmental impacts. Agreements such as the Paris Agreement represent an important step, but it is fundamental that they are strengthened and fulfilled with greater ambition. In addition, partnerships between governments, companies, non-governmental organizations, and civil society are fundamental to drive technological innovations and transform outdated economic models into sustainable alternatives.

Although the primary responsibility for implementing climate policies lies with governments and large corporations, individuals can also play a significant role in the fight against climate change. Small changes in lifestyle, such as reducing meat consumption, opting for less polluting means of transport, reducing food waste, and supporting companies committed to sustainability, can have a significant impact when adopted on a large scale. Awareness and active participation in environmental initiatives, such as reforestation projects or movements for climate justice, are effective ways to contribute to building a more balanced future.

Addressing climate change requires more than technological solutions; it requires a profound transformation in the way we interact with the planet and with each other. Holism teaches us that everything is interconnected and that every action has broad and lasting consequences. By adopting an integrated vision, which respects the limits of nature and promotes social justice, we can build a more sustainable and harmonious future for the next generations.

The complexity of global challenges demands a continuous commitment and coordinated action between individuals, communities, and nations. There are no simple or unique solutions, but a set of interconnected strategies that should be applied in a complementary manner. The transition to a sustainable world involves the strengthening of effective public policies, technological innovation aligned with environmental regeneration, and the development of an economy that prioritizes collective well-being without compromising natural resources.

In addition, addressing environmental and social crises requires a profound change in the prevailing mentality. Instead of seeing nature as an obstacle to growth, we must recognize it as an indispensable ally for the survival of humanity. This means rethinking our habits, values, and consumption relations, seeking models based on cooperation and equity. The culture of illusory abundance needs to give way to a paradigm of respect and responsibility, where every choice is made considering its long-term impacts.

The future depends on the decisions we make in the present. Every step forward in the fight against climate change, every initiative for ecological restoration, and every transformation in the way we produce and consume are fundamental to ensuring a more resilient and balanced world. If we learn from the mistakes of the past and adopt a genuine commitment to sustainability, we can face global challenges with intelligence and courage, ensuring that future generations inherit a habitable, diverse, and thriving planet.

Chapter 11
The Holistic Mind

The human mind manifests as a dynamic field of interactions between the body, emotions, thoughts, and subtle dimensions of existence, functioning as an integrated and interdependent system. For centuries, different philosophical and scientific traditions have attempted to comprehend its complexity, sometimes fragmenting its aspects, sometimes seeking a unified vision. With advances in psychology and neuroscience, it has become evident that reducing the mind to isolated processes does not capture its true essence. A holistic approach, on the other hand, recognizes that mental phenomena cannot be understood in a way dissociated from the body, the environment, and even spiritual aspects. This expanded conception allows for a deeper understanding of human behavior, emotions, and states of consciousness, broadening horizons in both academic research and therapeutic practices.

By integrating knowledge from psychology, biology, philosophy, and even spiritual traditions, it becomes clear that the mind does not operate in isolation within the brain but rather as a network of interactions between the nervous system, the body, and external reality. Stress, for example, does not only affect the emotional state but physically impacts the organism, altering brain chemistry, the immune system, and even gene expression. Similarly, practices such as meditation, conscious breathing, and physical exercise can modify neural patterns and promote states of deep well-being. This interconnection demonstrates that mental health cannot be treated only with reductionist methods but requires an integrative approach that takes into account multiple dimensions of human existence.

Furthermore, consciousness, seen by some currents as an emergent phenomenon of brain interactions, is approached by holistic perspectives as a broader manifestation, transcending the physical limits of the brain. Theorists suggest that the mind is not confined to neuronal activity but may be connected to a wider field of collective information and influences. This understanding aligns with discoveries in quantum physics, which indicate that reality can be influenced by perception and the interaction between observer and observed object. Thus, understanding the mind under a holistic view not only expands the frontiers of traditional psychology but also opens possibilities for new forms of self-knowledge, emotional balance, and human development.

The holistic view of the mind starts from the principle that the physical, emotional, mental, and spiritual aspects of the human being cannot be analyzed separately, as they are deeply interconnected and mutually influence each other. This understanding leads us to realize that a shaken emotional state can trigger physical manifestations, such as headaches, muscle tension, or digestive problems, just as practices aimed at physical well-being, such as regular exercise and a balanced diet, can positively impact mood and mental health.

This approach contrasts with the traditional reductionist view, which tends to treat the mind and body as separate entities, focusing only on isolated symptoms and neglecting their multifactorial origin. Holistic psychology, on the other hand, seeks to integrate these dimensions, recognizing that human well-being depends on the balance between body, mind, and spirit. This understanding has led to the development of more comprehensive therapeutic practices, which combine different approaches to treat the individual in their totality.

Within this context, humanistic psychology and transpersonal psychology emerge as branches that adopt this broader view of the mind and human experience. Humanistic psychology, driven by figures such as Abraham Maslow and Carl Rogers, emphasizes the importance of self-realization and the development of human potential, recognizing that each individual is unique and that the search for meaning and purpose is essential for well-being. At its core, this approach values the human capacity for growth, emphasizing empathy, authenticity, and personal development.

Transpersonal psychology, in turn, goes further, incorporating spiritual and transcendental aspects of human experience. It investigates expanded states of consciousness, exploring phenomena such as meditation, mystical experiences, and deep insights that transcend the limits of the individual ego and connect the human being to a broader dimension of existence. Researchers like Stanislav Grof and Ken Wilber have contributed significantly to this approach, demonstrating that the mind can be understood at different levels of consciousness and that spiritual experiences should not be dismissed as mere hallucinations but recognized as legitimate and transformative experiences.

Consciousness, one of the great mysteries of science and philosophy, is another fundamental aspect of the holistic approach. What is consciousness? How does it arise? What is its role in the universe? The holistic view suggests that consciousness is not a simple product of brain activity but an emerging phenomenon that results from the complex interaction between brain, body, and environment. According to some theorists, such as David Bohm and Rupert Sheldrake, consciousness may be a fundamental principle of the universe, permeating all levels of reality. This perspective aligns with many spiritual traditions that see consciousness as the basis of everything that exists, suggesting that the human mind is not confined to the brain but connects to a wider field of collective information and influences.

In practice, holistic psychology offers concrete applications in various areas, from therapy to education and personal development. In the therapeutic field, the holistic approach seeks to integrate different techniques, combining elements of cognitive-behavioral therapy, body therapy, meditation, and even spiritual practices to treat the individual as a whole. This view recognizes that psychological problems often have deep roots that go beyond the mental sphere, and may be linked to emotional imbalances, body patterns, and even energetic aspects.

One of the most effective tools within this paradigm is the practice of mindfulness and meditation, which has become widely recognized for its benefits in promoting well-being and mental clarity. Mindfulness helps in emotional regulation, reduces stress, and improves quality of life by helping the individual connect with the present moment and integrate their experiences more consciously.

In the educational field, holistic education is concerned not only with the transmission of academic knowledge but also with the integral development of the human being, taking into account cognitive, emotional, social, and spiritual aspects. This approach encourages creativity, empathy, and ecological awareness, preparing individuals for a more balanced and meaningful life.

In personal development, the holistic focus encourages the search for self-knowledge and spiritual growth, recognizing that true well-being is not limited to the absence of diseases, but involves a life aligned with inner values, purposes, and healthy relationships. Strategies such as the practice of gratitude, the strengthening of emotional resilience, and the cultivation of meaningful relationships are part of this journey towards balance and personal fulfillment.

Beyond the individual aspect, consciousness also manifests collectively. The so-called collective consciousness refers to the beliefs, values, and attitudes shared by a group or society, shaping behaviors and influencing social changes. This concept, developed by sociologists like Émile Durkheim, suggests that the human mind does not operate in isolation but is immersed in a collective field of influences and interactions. This perspective is supported by contemporary phenomena, such as the expansion of collective intelligence made possible by the internet and social networks, where groups of individuals collaborate to solve complex problems and promote global transformations.

However, the adoption of holistic psychology still faces challenges, especially due to resistance to change within some academic circles and the need for greater scientific validation for certain approaches. Even so, the growing awareness of the importance of integral well-being has driven a demand for more integrated and comprehensive practices. The intersection between science and spirituality, previously seen as a field of contradictions, has been progressively explored, opening new possibilities for understanding the mind and consciousness. Research in neuroscience, quantum physics, and transpersonal psychology continues to expand our perspectives, suggesting that the future of psychology may be increasingly interdisciplinary and holistic.

In this way, understanding the mind under a holistic perspective allows us to access a more complete view of human nature and its interconnection with the whole. By recognizing that body, mind, and spirit are parts of the same system, we are invited to develop a more integrated approach to life, promoting not only personal balance but also a more conscious and harmonious society.

This understanding broadens the way we deal with individual and collective challenges, encouraging practices that promote a state of greater internal and external coherence. When we adopt a holistic view, we realize that personal transformation does not occur in isolation but reverberates in relationships, culture, and even the way we interact with the environment. The awareness of this interconnectivity leads us to seek paths that integrate traditional and scientific knowledge, respecting the complexity of human experience and its multiple dimensions.

Furthermore, the adoption of a broader view of the mind and consciousness strengthens innovative approaches to mental health, education, and human development. Techniques that combine science and spirituality, such as integrative therapies and educational methodologies that value emotional intelligence and creativity, become increasingly relevant. This movement points to a future where knowledge will not be fragmented but articulated in a more systemic way, respecting the plurality of perspectives and the richness of human experiences.

Thus, the holistic mind is not just a theoretical concept, but an invitation to the practice of a more conscious and balanced living. By integrating body, emotions, and spirit into a single flow of experience, we cultivate not only personal well-being but also a positive impact on the world around us. This path invites us to recognize that true human growth is not only in the accumulation of information, but in the ability to live with presence, purpose, and harmony.

Chapter 12
Medicina Holística e Bem-Estar

Human health transcends the simple absence of disease, encompassing a dynamic balance between body, mind and environment. Throughout history, different medical systems have tried to explain and treat the functioning of the organism, often in a fragmented way. However, the holistic approach to health proposes an integrated vision, where physical, emotional, social and spiritual factors interact to promote or compromise well-being. This concept broadens the horizons of conventional medicine, recognizing that the internal and external balance of an individual is decisive for their quality of life. Thus, understanding health from this perspective allows not only to treat diseases, but also to act in the prevention and strengthening of human vitality.

Holistic medicine considers that each person is a unique system, with specific needs that go beyond the symptoms manifested in the body. Instead of just suppressing signs of diseases, this approach seeks to identify and treat the underlying causes of imbalances, promoting self-regulation and the natural healing of the organism. For this, it integrates traditional and contemporary practices, such as functional nutrition, energy therapies, phytotherapy, mindfulness and activities that favor emotional balance. This broader view of health also emphasizes the role of the patient as an active agent in their own well-being, encouraging healthy habits and a lifestyle aligned with the needs of the body and mind.

In addition to individual aspects, holistic health considers the interconnection of the human being with their environment and their community. The quality of air, water, food and social relationships directly influences the state of health, making essential an approach that goes beyond the isolated organism. In this context, practices such as integrative medicine, which combines conventional treatments with complementary therapies, have gained space in hospitals and health centers around the world. This fusion of knowledge demonstrates that science and tradition can coexist, bringing benefits both for the prevention and treatment of diseases. By adopting this perspective, the understanding of what it means to be truly healthy is broadened, promoting not only longevity, but also a fuller and more balanced life.

The principles of holistic medicine are fundamental to understand this integral approach to health, which goes beyond the simple elimination of symptoms and seeks harmony between body, mind and spirit. One of the essential pillars of this practice is the integral vision of the human being. Different from traditional medicine, which often focuses on isolated parts of the body, holistic medicine recognizes that all dimensions of the being are interconnected. This means that a physical problem may have emotional or spiritual origins and, in the same way, imbalances in the mind can manifest in diseases in the body. Thus, a person's health depends directly on the interaction and balance between these aspects, making it essential to look at the individual as a whole, and not just at their specific complaints.

In addition to this comprehensive view, holistic medicine emphasizes prevention and health promotion as essential aspects. Instead of acting only in the treatment of already manifested diseases, this approach seeks to prevent imbalances from happening. For this, it encourages healthy habits, such as a balanced diet, the regular practice of physical activities, relaxation techniques and effective strategies to deal with stress. Small changes in the routine, such as sleeping well, connecting with nature and cultivating positive thoughts, can have a profound impact on overall health. This preventive perspective not only improves the quality of life, but also reduces the need for invasive medical interventions, becoming a sustainable and beneficial approach in the long term.

Another central principle of holistic medicine is the individualization of treatment. Each person has a unique life history, with genetic predispositions, emotional experiences and distinct environmental conditions. For this reason, instead of following a fixed protocol, holistic medicine adapts treatments to the specific needs of each individual. What works for one person may not be suitable for another, and understanding this singularity is essential to achieve effective results. This personalization may involve adjustments in the diet, the choice of appropriate complementary therapies or even changes in the lifestyle that align with the individual characteristics of each patient.

Within this approach, the belief in the body's natural healing capacity is another essential point. The human organism has intrinsic mechanisms of self-regulation and regeneration, and holistic medicine seeks to stimulate these natural processes. Instead of relying exclusively on synthetic drugs, this vision values more natural methods, such as functional nutrition, the use of medicinal plants, energy therapies and physical activities that promote well-being. The idea is not to reject conventional medicine, but to integrate it with practices that respect the rhythm and nature of the body.

Furthermore, holistic medicine promotes a partnership relationship between the patient and the therapist. Different from the traditional approach, where the doctor dictates a treatment and the patient follows passively, in holistic medicine the patient assumes an active role in their own healing process. The therapist acts as a guide, helping the person to understand their body, their emotions and their patterns of behavior so that they can make healthier choices aligned with their well-being. This involvement makes the patient more aware of their health and responsible for their own balance, which strengthens the results of the adopted practices.

To achieve this integral well-being, holistic medicine combines a wide variety of therapeutic practices, each with a specific role in promoting health. Holistic nutrition, for example, starts from the principle that food not only serves to provide energy, but also directly influences the functioning of the organism and emotional health. A natural diet, rich in fruits, vegetables, whole grains and high-quality proteins, strengthens the immune system and contributes to the prevention of diseases. In addition, holistic nutrition takes into account the individual needs of each person, personalizing diets to treat specific conditions, such as inflammations, digestive disorders and hormonal imbalances.

Body therapies also play a crucial role in holistic medicine. Techniques such as massage therapy, chiropractic, osteopathy and acupuncture help to relieve tensions, improve blood circulation and restore the body's energy balance. These therapies recognize that physical well-being is directly linked to emotions and mental state, promoting relaxation and stress reduction. Acupuncture, for example, is based on the concept of vital energy that circulates through the body and, through the stimulation of specific points, can restore energy flow and alleviate various conditions, from muscle pain to emotional disorders.

Energy medicine is another relevant practice within the holistic approach. Methods such as Reiki, pranic healing and crystal therapy work with the body's subtle energy to restore balance and strengthen vitality. These therapies believe that energy imbalances can result in physical and emotional illnesses, and by rebalancing these flows, it is possible to promote a deep sense of well-being and harmony.

In addition to physical and energy therapies, holistic medicine also values mental and emotional practices. Methods such as psychotherapy, hypnotherapy and emotional freedom techniques (EFT) help people to deal with traumas, anxiety and negative thought patterns that affect their overall health. The impact of emotions on physical health is widely recognized, and taking care of the mind is an essential step to achieve an integral balance.

Spiritual practices are also part of this path of healing and well-being. Meditation, yoga, prayer and other forms of connection with the inner self help to cultivate mental peace, emotional clarity and a deeper sense of purpose. Many studies point out that these practices reduce stress levels, strengthen immunity and increase longevity, becoming valuable tools for a fuller life.

Holistic medicine is not opposed to conventional medicine, but seeks a balanced integration between the two approaches. For example, a patient with cancer can benefit from chemotherapy and radiotherapy, but can also adopt holistic therapies, such as acupuncture to alleviate side effects, meditation to reduce stress and a functional diet to strengthen the immune system. This fusion of knowledge provides a more complete and effective treatment, addressing not only physical needs, but also emotional and spiritual needs of the patient.

Self-care is also a fundamental pillar of holistic medicine. Small daily habits, such as maintaining a balanced diet, practicing exercises regularly, sleeping well, managing stress and cultivating healthy social connections, are essential for maintaining health and well-being. Self-care is not limited to the body, but also involves attention to emotions and spirituality, encouraging practices such as gratitude, reflection on life and the search for a meaningful purpose.

Despite the countless benefits of holistic medicine, there are still challenges to overcome. The lack of regulation in some practices and the skepticism on the part of sectors of conventional medicine are obstacles that limit the dissemination of this approach. However, as new scientific research validates the benefits of practices such as meditation, acupuncture and phytotherapy, the acceptance of holistic medicine grows, becoming an increasingly recognized complementary alternative.

In the end, holistic medicine offers us a comprehensive view of health, which considers the interconnection between body, mind and spirit. By adopting this approach, we can not only treat diseases, but also prevent imbalances and live with more harmony and fullness. More than a healing system, this medicine invites us to a journey of self-knowledge and integral care, promoting a healthier and more balanced life.

By recognizing the interdependence between the different aspects of human existence, holistic medicine teaches us that true well-being goes beyond the absence of diseases and manifests itself in the harmony between body, mind and spirit. This integrative look invites each individual to assume an active role in the care of their own health, adopting practices that strengthen not only physical vitality, but also emotional balance and connection with something greater. In this way, the journey to a healthy life becomes a continuous process of learning, self-knowledge and transformation.

The advancement of holistic medicine does not mean the replacement of traditional models, but rather the construction of a broader and complementary approach, where different forms of knowledge dialogue to provide more effective and humane treatments. The fusion between science and ancestral wisdom reinforces that healing should not be seen only as a mechanical act of repairing the body, but as a deep process of restoring the totality of the being. With this, a path opens for a more sensitive and personalized medicine, which respects the uniqueness of each individual and seeks to meet their needs completely.

By reconnecting with our own nature and understanding health from this integrative perspective, we realize that self-care and balance are daily practices that transcend the simple pursuit of longevity. Holistic medicine invites us to a life of greater presence, consciousness and well-being, in which health becomes not only an objective, but a reflection of the way we choose to live.

Chapter 13
Forming Complete Human Beings

Education is a transformative process that goes beyond the mere transmission of information and cognitive development. It is a path to the integral formation of the human being, involving not only the intellect but also the emotional, social, and spiritual dimensions. In the traditional model, the focus is often restricted to memorization of content and academic performance, neglecting fundamental aspects such as creativity, empathy, and emotional intelligence. However, a broader and more integrative approach allows learning to be meaningful, connected to reality, and promotes complete human development. Holistic education emerges as a response to this need, recognizing that each individual is unique and that true learning should encompass multiple dimensions of existence.

This educational perspective considers that knowledge cannot be dissociated from experience, and that the formation of the individual should include understanding oneself, interpersonal relationships, and the world around them. Instead of a standardized model centered solely on the acquisition of technical skills, holistic education values curiosity, autonomy, and the student's connection with learning. It encourages active methods such as interdisciplinary projects, artistic practices, meditation, and contact with nature, creating an environment conducive to the student discovering their potential in a genuine and authentic way.

This educational model also emphasizes the importance of human values, promoting cooperation, compassion, and social responsibility, preparing individuals not only for the job market but for a full and conscious life.

In addition to transforming the way knowledge is transmitted, holistic education also proposes a new vision of the role of the educator. They should not only be a transmitter of content but a facilitator of learning, someone who inspires, guides, and motivates students to explore the world with critical thinking and creativity. For this, it is essential that the educator themselves are committed to their personal development and with a reflective stance, open to new approaches and methodologies.

By integrating scientific, philosophical, and cultural knowledge, holistic education not only expands the possibilities of learning but also contributes to the construction of a more balanced world in which knowledge serves as a means for human and collective flourishing.

Holistic education is structured on fundamental principles that shape its integral and humanized approach. The first of these is the integral vision of the human being, which recognizes the interconnection between body, mind, and spirit. This principle proposes a development that goes beyond the intellect, encompassing emotional, social, and spiritual dimensions, understanding that true learning occurs when there is balance between these aspects. From this vision, teaching ceases to be fragmented and begins to connect with the individual's experience and growth, allowing each student to develop in their totality.

Another essential aspect is respect for individuality. Each human being has their own talents, rhythms, and ways of learning. Holistic education values these differences and seeks to personalize teaching so that it meets the specific needs of each student. Instead of imposing a single teaching model, this approach allows learning to happen naturally, respecting curiosity and individual interests. Thus, educators act as guides, helping students discover their own passions and potentialities.

Meaningful learning also occupies a central role in this model. Teaching should not be a mechanical accumulation of information but a living experience connected to reality. When knowledge makes sense and is related to the students' daily lives, it becomes more solid and lasting. Therefore, holistic education emphasizes methods that promote creativity, inquiry, and critical thinking, allowing students to construct knowledge in an active and participatory way.

In addition to cognitive development, holistic education prioritizes the construction of values and attitudes that promote individual and collective well-being. Empathy, cooperation, social responsibility, and respect for nature are fundamental pillars of this process.

Learning is not limited to the assimilation of concepts but includes the formation of ethical and conscious citizens capable of contributing to a more balanced and sustainable world. This principle reinforces the idea that education should not only prepare for the job market but for life as a whole.

The connection with the community and the world further broadens this perspective. Holistic education recognizes that the individual is not an isolated entity but part of a larger system. Thus, it encourages active participation in local and global issues, stimulating a sense of belonging and responsibility. Community projects, outdoor activities, and discussions on social and environmental themes are part of this approach, promoting a broad and integrative worldview.

To realize these principles, holistic education adopts several practices that aim to promote more complete development. Project-based learning is one of them. Instead of studying subjects in isolation, students carry out interdisciplinary projects that connect different areas of knowledge. This methodology favors the practical application of learned concepts, encouraging skills such as problem-solving, teamwork, and creativity. A project can involve the creation of a documentary about sustainability, the development of an educational application, or the organization of a science fair. In this way, students learn in a dynamic and engaging way.

Emotional education is also an essential component. The development of emotional intelligence allows students to understand and manage their emotions, promoting well-being and healthy relationships. Practices such as meditation and mindfulness are incorporated into daily school life to help with self-control and concentration. In addition, activities that encourage self-expression, such as conversation circles and reflective writing, allow students to develop greater awareness about themselves and others.

Concern for the environment is also present in holistic education, through ecological education. This principle seeks to develop environmental awareness from an early age, encouraging connection with nature and the adoption of sustainable practices. Students are encouraged to plant gardens, recycle materials, participate in conservation projects, and carry out outdoor activities. This experience strengthens respect for the environment and awakens ecological responsibility, preparing citizens more aware of the importance of sustainability.

Art and creativity play a fundamental role in this educational model. Artistic expression allows students to explore their imagination, develop their sensitivity, and find unique forms of communication. Music, dance, theater, painting, and creative writing are powerful tools to stimulate self-knowledge and experimentation. By including artistic activities in the curriculum, holistic education enables students to connect with their emotions and acquire a more sensitive view of the world.

Another important pillar is education for peace, which seeks to develop skills for peaceful conflict resolution and promote respect for diversity. In a world marked by social and cultural challenges, this approach teaches students to deal with differences constructively. Techniques such as conflict mediation, intercultural dialogue, and empathy exercises are applied to create a more harmonious and cooperative environment.

For this approach to be effective, the role of the holistic educator needs to be reassessed. The teacher is not only a transmitter of knowledge but a facilitator of learning. They must create a welcoming environment where students feel comfortable to explore, question, and learn autonomously. In addition, it is essential that the educator themselves are in constant development, both professionally and personally. Reflective practice is essential to improve their methodologies and so that they also experience the principles of holistic education in their own lives.

Despite the numerous benefits, the implementation of this approach faces challenges. Resistance to change is one of the main obstacles since the traditional teaching model is deeply rooted in society. In addition, the lack of resources and support in some institutions hinders the adoption of innovative practices. However, the growing interest in alternative teaching methods has created opportunities to expand holistic education.

Technology and globalization also play an important role in this scenario. Access to online platforms, courses, and collaboration networks facilitates the exchange of experiences between educators and students, allowing holistic education to reach an increasingly wider audience. These tools expand the possibilities of learning and help overcome geographical and structural barriers.

Thus, holistic education presents itself as a path to the formation of complete human beings, prepared to deal with the challenges of the world in a conscious and balanced way. By integrating different dimensions of knowledge and valuing individuality, this approach transforms teaching into a more meaningful and enriching experience. More than a pedagogical model, holistic education is an invitation to a learning that respects the essence of each individual and promotes a full and harmonious development.

By adopting this approach, education becomes a living process that respects individual rhythms and favors the construction of a more empathetic and sustainable world. Instead of forming only professionals trained for the market, holistic education cultivates complete human beings, prepared to face challenges with sensitivity, creativity, and responsibility. This transformation is not limited to the classroom but extends to society, impacting the way we relate, work, and collaborate for a more balanced future.

The application of this model requires structural and cultural changes, but small steps can already generate great impacts. Schools, educators, and families that incorporate elements of holistic education contribute to a more welcoming and meaningful environment for new generations. When children and young people are encouraged to express their uniqueness, value their emotions, and connect with their purpose, they become more fulfilled and aware adults of the role they play in the world.

Thus, the formation of complete human beings is not only a pedagogical ideal but a commitment to the integral development of humanity. When learning expands beyond the limits of technical knowledge and embraces the totality of human experience, we create not only more prepared individuals but a more just, balanced, and connected society with the essential values of life.

Chapter 14
Expressions of Totality

Art and creativity are essential manifestations of human experience, acting as bridges between the inner world and external reality. Far beyond mere aesthetic expressions, they represent a channel of deep communication, capable of translating emotions, ideas and perceptions that often escape the limitations of verbal language. From the first records of humanity, such as cave paintings and mythological narratives, to the most modern forms of digital and interactive art, creativity has been a vital force for understanding and transforming the world. When we engage in the creative act—whether through painting, music, writing, dancing or any other form of expression—we experience a state of full presence, in which body, mind and spirit align, promoting a feeling of connection and belonging to the totality of existence.

Artistic creation and creative thinking are not skills restricted to talented or trained individuals, but rather potentialities inherent to all human beings. Creativity manifests itself in the way we solve problems, how we adapt to changes and how we interact with the environment around us. In an increasingly fast-paced and mechanized world, recovering creative freedom is essential to restore emotional and spiritual balance. Artistic practice, in addition to offering a means of self-expression, functions as a powerful therapeutic tool, helping in the understanding of repressed feelings, in overcoming internal challenges and in the construction of a state of integral well-being. When we allow ourselves to explore and expand our creativity, we activate a transforming force that impacts not only our own existence, but also the relationships we establish and society as a whole.

In addition to individual impact, art and creativity have a fundamental role in the collective evolution of humanity. They allow us to transcend cultural barriers, stimulate dialogue between different perspectives and foster a broader and more inclusive vision of the world. Art has historically been a reflection of the concerns and aspirations of each era, functioning as an agent of questioning and social change. When allied with innovation, creativity also drives scientific discoveries, technological advances and new forms of social organization, contributing to the construction of more harmonious and sustainable realities. In this way, by nurturing creativity and artistic expression in our daily lives, we not only enrich our personal journey, but also actively participate in the continuous process of creation and renewal of the world that surrounds us.

Art, in its essence, transcends the barriers of verbal communication, allowing emotions, ideas and experiences to be expressed in a deep and meaningful way. Every stroke of a painting, every note of a melody and every movement of a dance carries with it a message that resonates beyond words. When we engage in artistic creation, we transcend the limitations of language and access a form of expression that connects the depths of our soul to the world around us. Art not only reflects our vision of the world, but also enables us to share it, becoming a link between individuality and the collective.

More than a simple aesthetic manifestation, art acts holistically, integrating different aspects of the human being. When we dance, our body moves in sync with deep emotions and, often, with a spiritual connection that transcends the present moment. Music, in turn, has the power to evoke long-held memories, awaken intense feelings and elevate our perception beyond materiality. Literature, through words, transports us to imaginary worlds, offering new perspectives and broadening our understanding of existence. Thus, each art form allows us to explore our totality, uniting body, mind and spirit in a unique experience of expression and connection.

Creativity, in turn, is a primordial force that permeates human existence. Far from being an exclusive gift of artists, it manifests itself in all of us, driving problem solving, innovation and the transformation of the world around us. Every decision we make, every solution found for a daily challenge, is an expression of this innate creative capacity. From a broader perspective, creativity connects us to a universal energy, a continuous flow of creation that shapes reality and allows us to interact with it in an active and innovative way.

When we allow ourselves to create, we align our consciousness with this flow, transcending the barriers of the ego and experiencing a state of unity and belonging to the whole. Creativity teaches us that there are no limits to imagination, and that reality can be constantly reinvented from new ideas and perspectives. It is this ability to see beyond the obvious that drives not only art, but also great scientific discoveries, technological advances and innovations that shape society.

In addition to being a tool of expression and innovation, art also plays an essential role in healing and emotional well-being. Art therapy, for example, uses the creative process as a means of exploring repressed feelings, processing traumas and promoting self-expression in a safe environment. People who find it difficult to verbalize their feelings often discover in art a powerful channel to understand and transform their emotions. Painting, drawing, sculpture and other forms of visual expression allow the psyche to manifest itself in a symbolic way, often revealing internal aspects that were hidden.

The artistic experience can also be compared to a meditative state. When we are deeply immersed in creation, we enter a flow where time seems to disappear, the mind quiets down and attention turns completely to the present. This state of full presence is similar to meditation, bringing benefits such as stress reduction, increased mental clarity and a deep sense of inner peace. By creating without judgment, without the pressure of a perfect end result, we allow art to flow naturally, becoming a mirror of our internal state and a path to personal transformation.

In the context of innovation, creativity becomes an essential element for the evolution of society. In a constantly changing world, the ability to think outside established patterns and find original solutions to complex problems is indispensable. Creativity applied to innovation is not restricted to the development of new technologies or products, but also extends to the way we structure organizations, conduct human relations and face global challenges. Creative thinking allows us to break with limiting paradigms, envision new possibilities and build a more balanced and sustainable future.

Holistic innovation, in turn, recognizes that contemporary challenges require interdisciplinary and integrated approaches. Environmental, social and economic problems are interconnected, and finding effective solutions requires a systemic vision that considers the complexity of these interactions. When we apply creativity holistically, we are encouraged to collaborate, to share knowledge and to develop strategies that promote well-being not only individual, but collective.

Art also has an intrinsic connection with spirituality. Many ancestral traditions have used and still use art as a means of expressing the sacred and establishing a bridge with the divine. Religious icons, mandalas, sculptures, songs and ritual dances are examples of artistic manifestations that transcend materiality and evoke a spiritual dimension. In various cultures, music is used in sacred ceremonies to elevate consciousness and facilitate states of ecstasy and communion with the transcendent.

Furthermore, the artistic experience itself can become a journey of self-knowledge and spiritual seeking. When we create or appreciate art, we often come across profound existential questions: What is the meaning of life? What is the nature of reality? What is our role in the universe? Art invites us to explore these mysteries without the need for definitive answers, allowing us to simply feel, experience and contemplate the vastness of existence.

It is important to remember that creativity is not restricted to formal arts. It can be cultivated in everyday life, in small actions that make life more vibrant and meaningful. Cooking a new recipe, decorating an environment in a unique way, writing a diary, improvising a melody on the guitar or simply finding a different way to solve a problem are expressions of creativity. By adopting a creative approach to life, we become more open to new experiences, more adaptable to changes and more aware of the beauty present in every moment.

Despite its importance, art and creativity still face challenges in many societies. The lack of incentive and the utilitarian view that privileges only productivity can lead to the devaluation of these essential manifestations. However, the growing recognition of the benefits of art for mental health, education and innovation has driven a greater appreciation of these practices. Today, technology has been a great ally in this process, democratizing access to art through digital platforms, social networks and creative tools that allow anyone to share their expression with the world.

In the end, art and creativity connect us to the totality of existence, allowing us to express, transform and understand life in ways that go beyond the intellect. They offer us a refuge of authenticity amidst the demands of modernity and remind us that we are, above all, creative beings. By embracing art and creativity in our daily lives, we find more meaning, joy and connection, contributing to the construction of a more harmonious and inspiring world.

By understanding art and creativity as expressions of totality, we recognize that they not only reflect our essence, but also allow us to shape and transform the reality around us. Artistic creation invites us to go beyond the limits of linear thinking and to explore new possibilities, awakening a sense of discovery and enchantment that rescues the richness of human experience. This process does not need to be linked to perfection or technique, but rather to authenticity, to the courage to express what pulsates within us and to the freedom to give form to the invisible.

When we cultivate creativity as a principle of life, we learn to see the world with a more attentive and sensitive eye, finding beauty and meaning in the small things of everyday life. Art teaches us to value the present moment, to reconnect with intuition and to open ourselves to the unexpected, allowing imagination to guide us to paths previously unimaginable. Thus, the act of creating ceases to be a privilege and becomes an inherent right to every human being, a constant invitation to reinvent oneself and to expand.

In the end, we realize that art not only gives color and form to life, but also reveals to us what we are in our essence. It connects us to the sacred, to the playful, to the mystery and to the truth that transcends words. Whether painting a canvas, composing a melody or simply reinventing our way of living, we express the totality of our being and become co-authors of the great work that is existence.

Chapter 15
Living in Harmony

Human connection is one of the most powerful forces shaping our existence, directly influencing our emotional, mental, and even physical health. From the earliest moments of life, the bonds we establish with others play an essential role in forming our identity and well-being. Neuroscience and psychology demonstrate that social interaction activates brain circuits fundamental to the development of empathy, resilience, and a sense of belonging. When we cultivate healthy relationships, we not only strengthen our emotions but also promote a deeper balance between mind and body. On the other hand, the lack of meaningful connections can lead to feelings of loneliness, stress, and imbalances that affect various areas of life.

From a holistic perspective, relationships go beyond superficial interactions and become opportunities for personal and collective growth. Every human encounter is a reflection of the interconnectedness of life, offering valuable lessons about ourselves and the world. When we relate with presence and authenticity, we create spaces of genuine exchange, where active listening, respect, and empathy become essential pillars. This approach helps us to see the challenges of relationships not as obstacles, but as opportunities to deepen our understanding of ourselves and others. Similarly, life in community is an extension of this process, promoting a sense of mutual responsibility and collaboration, fundamental to the construction of more balanced and harmonious societies.

Beyond individual impact, interpersonal connection influences the social structure and evolution of communities. When relationships are guided by values such as compassion and cooperation, support networks are created that can transform challenges into collective opportunities. The union of different perspectives and talents generates innovation, strengthens resilience, and expands the sense of belonging, essential elements for the sustainable development of societies. In an increasingly globalized and digital world, cultivating meaningful relationships and nurturing the community spirit are attitudes that promote well-being and enrich the human journey. Thus, by recognizing the importance of relationships in building a fuller life, we can transform our interactions into sources of growth, harmony, and true connection.

Relationships are the essence of human experience, directly influencing our way of living and perceiving the world around us. From the first bonds formed in childhood, whether with family or caregivers, to the friendships and romantic relationships we cultivate throughout life, all these connections shape our identity, providing emotional support and strengthening our self-esteem. Human contact, more than a social need, is a foundation for personal growth, providing valuable learning and allowing us to explore our own essence through the other.

From a holistic perspective, relationships transcend simple daily coexistence. Each interaction is an opportunity to evolve emotionally and spiritually, because, by relating to different people, we are challenged to broaden our worldview, develop empathy, and practice compassion. Community life, in turn, represents this same dynamic on a larger scale, where the sharing of experiences, challenges, and achievements strengthens the collective structure, promoting balance and well-being.

The need for human connection is rooted in our biology. Research shows that prolonged isolation can have severe adverse effects, increasing the risks of mental and physical illness. In contrast, maintaining healthy relationships contributes to longevity and quality of life. However, true connection goes beyond physical presence; it requires genuine involvement, willingness to listen attentively, and the sincere desire to understand the other. When we feel valued for who we really are, our self-confidence is strengthened, creating a positive cycle that impacts both ourselves and those around us.

In this context, the community emerges as an essential space for the development and sustenance of these relationships. It represents a circle of support where each individual finds belonging and security to share experiences, exchange knowledge, and face challenges collectively. Cooperation within a community strengthens the bonds between its members, creating an environment of trust and mutual respect. During periods of difficulty, this support network becomes even more fundamental, because solidarity among individuals is what enables the overcoming of adversities.

Empathy and compassion play a central role in building deep bonds. Empathy allows us to feel and understand the emotions of others, while compassion drives us to act to alleviate the suffering of the other. When practiced consciously, these qualities promote more harmonious and resolving relationships. They facilitate communication, making us more open to different perspectives and more skilled in conflict resolution. In a world full of challenges, cultivating these virtues can transform not only our individual interactions, but the entire social dynamic.

Collaboration and cooperation are essential for the functioning of relationships and community life. When we work together towards a common goal, we recognize the value of each contribution and learn to respect differences. In a holistic approach, this exchange becomes even more meaningful, because it reveals that each person has unique skills and perspectives that enrich the group as a whole. By embracing diversity as a valuable resource, we create more inclusive, innovative, and strengthened environments.

However, relationships and living in community are not always free of challenges. Conflicts and misunderstandings are inevitable, as each individual carries with them different experiences, beliefs, and values. The important thing is not to avoid these difficulties, but to learn to face them constructively. The healthy resolution of conflicts involves open and honest communication, active listening, and the willingness to see the situation from different perspectives. Dialogue and mediation are powerful tools to transform misunderstandings into learning, strengthening bonds instead of breaking them.

Spirituality can be a transforming element in relationships and community life. It teaches us to see others as part of a larger network, connected by something beyond individuality. When we incorporate this vision, we begin to value relationships more, practicing gratitude, respect, and mutual care. Practices such as meditation, prayer, and community service help to nurture these connections, creating a sense of shared purpose and meaning that strengthens interpersonal bonds.

With globalization and the advancement of technology, the notion of community has expanded beyond geographical boundaries. Today, we interact with people from different cultures, traditions, and perspectives, which challenges us to broaden our understanding of humanity as a whole. The global community reminds us of our interdependence and invites us to cooperate to solve challenges that affect everyone, such as climate change, social inequality, and humanitarian crises. By adopting a more conscious and supportive stance, we can contribute to a more balanced and sustainable world.

Relationships and community life are fundamental pillars for human well-being and evolution.

They offer us emotional support, a sense of belonging, and constant opportunities for learning and growth. By cultivating empathy, compassion, and collaboration, we strengthen not only our personal bonds, but also the social fabric as a whole. Thus, we can transform our daily interactions into sources of harmony and evolution, contributing to a fairer and more connected world.

Living in harmony does not mean the absence of challenges, but the willingness to face them with maturity, understanding, and respect. The construction of authentic relationships requires an attentive look at the other, but also at ourselves, because only by cultivating an internal balance can we interact healthily with those around us. This journey involves self-knowledge, openness to dialogue, and the ability to recognize both our strengths and our limitations, allowing human coexistence to become a space of mutual growth.

As we strengthen our bonds, we also broaden our vision of the impact we have on the world. Small gestures of kindness, patience, and cooperation generate waves of influence that go beyond our immediate circle, reverberating in the community and society as a whole. When we understand that every connection is an opportunity for learning and exchange, we become agents of transformation, contributing to a more welcoming and balanced environment.

In the end, the harmony we seek outside begins within us. The daily practice of empathy, respect, and cooperation teaches us that living well is not just an individual issue, but a collective process of building a more conscious and humane world. By nurturing relationships based on authenticity and care, we not only find more meaning in our own journey, but also inspire others to do the same, weaving, together, a network of true and transforming connections.

Chapter 16
Beyond Material Growth

Contemporary economics is undergoing a moment of fundamental transformation, in which the pursuit of material growth can no longer be the sole objective of societies. For decades, economic development was measured almost exclusively by the increase in Gross Domestic Product (GDP), an indicator that, although useful, does not fully reflect the quality of life of the population or the health of ecosystems. The limitation of this approach has become evident in the face of global challenges such as climate change, social inequality, and the depletion of natural resources. The need for a new economic paradigm, which considers human well-being and environmental sustainability as central pillars, has become increasingly urgent. Faced with this scenario, holistic economics emerges as an innovative alternative, proposing an integrated vision that balances development, social equity, and environmental preservation. This approach suggests that economic progress should be redefined, incorporating metrics that go beyond material growth, including people's happiness, the equitable distribution of wealth, and the regeneration of ecosystems.

To fully understand holistic economics, it is essential to recognize the interdependence between the economic, social, and environmental systems. Unlike the traditional model, which sees the economy as an isolated and autonomous entity, holistic economics considers that prosperity depends on multiple and interconnected factors. A truly prosperous economy is not one that only generates wealth, but one that also guarantees quality of life, access to essential services, and equitable opportunities for all individuals. Furthermore, holistic economics proposes a change in the way resources are used and distributed, encouraging practices that minimize waste and promote responsible use of natural assets. The concept of "growth at any cost" is replaced by a regenerative development model, in which economic activity not only avoids damage to the environment but actively contributes to its restoration. In this way, this approach not only responds to environmental and social crises but also offers a path to a more resilient and sustainable future.

Adopting a holistic economy requires a profound revision of economic systems and public policies. The transition to this model involves structural changes that include the creation of new indicators of progress, the implementation of policies that encourage the circular and regenerative economy, and the strengthening of economic models that promote equity and democratic participation. Companies and governments play a fundamental role in this transformation, but individuals also have a significant impact. Small changes, such as conscious consumption, support for local businesses, and the adoption of sustainable practices in daily life, can generate multiplier effects that drive this new economy. Awareness and education are essential tools in this process, as they allow society to understand the benefits of this approach and actively engage in building a fairer and more balanced future. Holistic economics, therefore, is not just an economic theory, but a new way of thinking and acting, oriented towards the creation of more sustainable, resilient, and humanized societies.

Holistic economics is based on essential principles that redefine the concept of progress, broadening its perspective beyond material growth. At its core, this approach recognizes that true human well-being cannot be measured only by the accumulation of wealth or by the increase in Gross Domestic Product (GDP), but by the quality of life of people, by environmental preservation, and by social justice. In this way, holistic economics integrates several fundamental pillars that guide its practice and application in the contemporary world.

The first of these pillars is the integral vision of well-being. Unlike traditional economics, which prioritizes economic growth as an end in itself, holistic economics understands that development must encompass a wide range of factors, including health, education, social relations, culture, and the environment. It starts from the principle that the prosperity of a society cannot be dissociated from the well-being of the people who make it up. Thus, instead of focusing only on increasing production and consumption, this approach seeks to ensure that individuals have access to decent living conditions, emotional balance, and active participation in the community.

Another essential principle is ecological sustainability, which recognizes that the economy does not exist in isolation but is deeply interconnected with ecosystems. The traditional model, based on the relentless exploitation of natural resources, has proven unsustainable, leading to the depletion of raw materials, the increase in pollution, and climate change. Holistic economics, on the other hand, proposes a more harmonious relationship between economic activity and the environment. Instead of just mitigating negative impacts, it promotes regenerative practices, which restore biodiversity, reduce waste, and ensure that natural resources are used in a balanced and conscious way, to preserve the quality of life of future generations.

Social justice and equity also occupy a central position in holistic economics. In a world marked by deep economic and social inequalities, this approach seeks to ensure that prosperity is distributed fairly and accessible to all. This means combating social exclusion, promoting public policies that reduce poverty, and creating mechanisms that guarantee equitable opportunities for all layers of society. In this context, practices such as the solidarity economy, which values cooperation and self-management, become fundamental for building a more inclusive and democratic economic model.

In addition, holistic economics values diversity and resilience. Instead of relying on a single sector or economic model, it encourages the creation of diverse and adaptable systems, which are capable of facing crises and unexpected changes. This includes strengthening local economies, stimulating innovation, and valuing traditional cultures and knowledge. Economic and cultural diversity makes societies more flexible and prepared to deal with challenges, ensuring that they can reinvent themselves in the face of global transformations.

Another essential aspect is participation and economic democracy. Holistic economics recognizes that economic decisions affect everyone's lives and, therefore, must be taken transparently and inclusively. This means encouraging the active participation of the population in the definition of economic policies and in the management of resources. Models of participatory governance, cooperatives, and social enterprises are examples of how this approach can be applied in practice, creating an environment where the economy is managed more fairly and collaboratively.

The implementation of holistic economics takes place through various practices that are already being adopted in different parts of the world. A significant example is the circular economy, a model that seeks to eliminate waste and maximize the reuse of resources. Unlike the traditional linear system – based on the logic of "extract, produce, discard" – the circular economy proposes a continuous cycle of reuse, in which materials and products are reintegrated into the production process, reducing the need to extract new resources and minimizing environmental impacts.

Another important approach within holistic economics is the solidarity economy, which is based on cooperation and social justice. This model values practices such as cooperatives, community banks, and local currencies, promoting economic inclusion and self-sufficiency of communities. By strengthening networks of mutual support and encouraging fair trade, the solidarity economy reduces inequalities and creates sustainable alternatives to the conventional economic system.

The well-being economy is also an essential component of this approach, as it redefines indicators of progress. Instead of measuring economic success only by GDP growth, this perspective considers metrics that reflect the quality of life of the population. Indicators such as the Gross National Happiness (GNH) and the Genuine Progress Indicator (GPI) take into account aspects such as health, education, environment, and psychological well-being, offering a more comprehensive view of human development.

The regenerative economy goes beyond simple sustainability, proposing practices that not only preserve but restore and revitalize ecosystems. This includes initiatives such as regenerative agriculture, which recovers soil fertility and promotes biodiversity, and environmental restoration projects, which help to reverse damage caused by human degradation. The central idea of this approach is that the economy can be a positive agent in the regeneration of the planet, and not just a factor of destruction.

In addition, the local and community economy plays a fundamental role in building a more balanced and resilient economic model. By encouraging local consumption and production, this approach strengthens small businesses, reduces dependence on global supply chains, and fosters a sense of belonging and cooperation within communities.

Technology and innovation also play a crucial role in holistic economics. Advances such as renewable energy, precision agriculture, and blockchain can be used to promote sustainability, inclusion, and efficiency. However, it is essential that technological development be guided by ethical principles and social responsibility, ensuring that its benefits are distributed equitably and that its environmental impacts are minimized.

Despite the numerous advantages, holistic economics faces significant challenges. Resistance to change, dependence on traditional economic systems, and lack of institutional support are obstacles that need to be overcome. However, the opportunities are vast. The growing interest in sustainability, the demand for fairer practices, and the expansion of global collaboration networks offer a favorable scenario for the consolidation of this new approach.

Individuals also play a fundamental role in the transition to holistic economics. Small changes in everyday life, such as adopting more conscious consumption, supporting local businesses, and participating in community initiatives, can generate significant impacts. Education and awareness are essential tools to drive this cultural transformation, creating a more informed society engaged in building a sustainable future.

In this way, holistic economics invites us to rethink the way we relate to the economy, the environment, and society. By adopting this perspective, we can build a world where progress is measured not only by material wealth but by collective well-being, by the regeneration of nature, and by social justice. This approach not only helps us face the challenges of the present but also inspires us to create a more harmonious, inclusive, and sustainable future.

The realization of holistic economics depends on the convergence of efforts between governments, companies, and citizens. For this transformation to occur effectively, it is necessary for public policies to be reformulated to prioritize regenerative economic models, guaranteeing incentives for sustainable practices and reducing dependence on predatory sectors. At the same time, companies need to assume a role of co-responsibility, adopting production and management models that respect environmental limits and promote social equity. However, no change will be truly lasting without the engagement of the population, which, through daily choices and active participation in political and economic processes, can strengthen this new vision of development.

More than a set of economic strategies, holistic economics represents a profound shift in the way society views progress. It challenges the logic of unlimited growth and proposes a new mentality based on the balance between prosperity and preservation, between innovation and respect for traditions, between individual and collective well-being. It is an invitation to re-evaluate our priorities and recognize that true wealth is not found only in the accumulation of goods, but in the quality of human relationships, in the health of ecosystems and in the ability to guarantee a dignified future for the next generations.

The path to implementing this model will not be simple, but the transformations already underway demonstrate that this change is not only possible, but necessary. Every step towards a fairer, more sustainable, and integrated economy strengthens the foundations for a more balanced and resilient world. As governments, businesses, and individuals become aware of the impact of their decisions, the possibility of building an economic system that values, above all, life in all its forms, grows. The challenge is launched: choose between the inertia of the past or the construction of a future in which prosperity and harmony go hand in hand.

Chapter 17
Systemic Visions for a Better World

Modern societies face increasingly complex and interconnected challenges, demanding political approaches that transcend fragmentation and immediate interests. Traditional governance, often guided by short electoral cycles and influences from power groups, struggles to address systemic problems like climate change, social inequality, and recurring economic crises. These challenges cannot be solved in isolation, as they are deeply intertwined and require a broad and integrated vision. Holistic politics and governance emerge as a necessary response to this gap, proposing a model that prioritizes the interconnection between different aspects of society, the active participation of the population, and long-term sustainability. Instead of reactive policies that only combat the symptoms of problems, this approach seeks to identify and treat their structural causes, promoting a balance between economic growth, social justice, and environmental preservation.

To build a more effective and sustainable political model, it is essential to rethink the foundations of governance, incorporating principles that favor evidence-based decisions, transparency, and equity.

Holistic politics recognizes that the prosperity of a nation cannot be measured only by economic growth, but also by the quality of life of its citizens, access to fundamental rights, and the health of ecosystems. This model emphasizes the need to broaden democratic processes, allowing different sectors of society to actively participate in decisions that affect them. This includes mechanisms of participatory democracy, such as collaborative budgets and popular assemblies, as well as the incorporation of traditional and scientific knowledge in the formulation of public policies. Furthermore, holistic governance values cooperation between different levels of government and sectors of society, promoting partnerships that strengthen the resilience of communities and ensure the implementation of effective and lasting solutions.

The transition to holistic governance is not without challenges, as it requires profound cultural, structural, and institutional changes. Resistance to the new, the influence of established interests, and the complexity of political systems are obstacles to be overcome. However, the advancement of technology and the growing global awareness of the need for more sustainable models create unprecedented opportunities for this transformation. Digital tools can increase transparency and citizen participation, while global collaboration networks facilitate the exchange of ideas and best practices between different countries and communities. The engagement of citizens is a crucial element in this process, as holistic politics is not built only from the top down, but also through daily actions that promote values such as justice, solidarity, and collective responsibility. By strengthening democratic participation and adopting an integrated vision of governance, it is possible to create more just, resilient, and prepared societies to face the challenges of the future.

Holistic politics and governance are based on principles that aim to transform the way societies face global challenges, promoting sustainable, fair, and participatory solutions. The first essential principle is the systemic vision, which recognizes the interconnection between issues such as climate change, social inequality, and loss of biodiversity. Instead of treating the symptoms of problems in isolation, this approach seeks to understand their structural causes, adopting strategies that consider the multiple factors that influence these phenomena. Thus, effective policies must take into account not only economic variables, but also social and environmental impacts, ensuring that short-term decisions do not compromise future sustainability.

Another fundamental pillar is participation and inclusion. Holistic governance argues that all sectors of society, including marginalized groups and local communities, should have an active voice in decision-making. This means valuing traditional and academic knowledge, ensuring that different perspectives are considered in the formulation of public policies. The adoption of mechanisms such as participatory budgets, popular consultations, and citizen assemblies strengthens democracy by providing greater representativeness and social engagement. In this way, government decisions cease to be the exclusivity of political and economic elites and begin to reflect, in a fairer way, the real needs of the population.

Sustainability and resilience are also central principles of holistic politics. Every decision must take into account its long-term impacts and the need to preserve natural resources for future generations. This implies not only environmental conservation, but also the creation of social and economic systems capable of adapting and resisting crises. The resilience of communities can be strengthened through economic diversification, environmental education, and policies that encourage regenerative practices, such as sustainable agriculture and the circular economy.

Justice and equity are other fundamental principles. Holistic governance seeks to reduce inequalities and ensure that everyone has access to opportunities and basic resources, such as education, health, and decent housing. This requires redistributive policies and a commitment to social inclusion, promoting collective well-being instead of concentrating benefits in small privileged groups. Measures such as progressive taxation, income transfer programs, and investments in social infrastructure are examples of how equity can be incorporated into public policies.

Finally, transparency and accountability are essential to ensure the integrity of institutions. Governments and organizations must be open, ethical, and accountable to society, avoiding corruption and promoting trust between citizens and political leaders.

Tools such as open data, public audits, and government monitoring platforms are mechanisms that can increase transparency and strengthen democracy.

Holistic politics and governance are not limited to abstract concepts; they translate into concrete practices that are already being implemented in various parts of the world. An example of this are evidence-based policies, which use scientific data and in-depth analysis to support government decisions. Instead of adopting impulsive measures or influenced by political interests, this model prioritizes solutions based on research and successful experiences. The consideration of social, environmental, and economic impacts before the implementation of public policies makes decisions more effective and aligned with the real needs of the population.

Another crucial aspect is multi-level governance, which recognizes the need for cooperation between different spheres of public power. Global problems require coordinated solutions between local, national, and international governments, as well as collaboration between the public, private, and civil society organizations. This approach fosters strategic partnerships and facilitates the implementation of integrated policies, strengthening the resilience of communities and promoting sustainable development.

Participatory democracy also plays a central role. Mechanisms such as participatory budgets, public consultations, and citizen assemblies allow the population to directly influence the decisions that affect their daily lives. By promoting greater civic involvement, this approach strengthens the legitimacy of public policies and reduces political alienation, encouraging a sense of collective responsibility in building the future.

In the environmental field, sustainability policies are fundamental to ensure the preservation of ecosystems and the mitigation of climate change. Governments that adopt the holistic perspective invest in renewable energies, energy efficiency, reforestation, and circular economy, seeking to minimize waste and environmental impacts. Incentives for companies and citizens to adopt sustainable practices are also part of this model, promoting a culture of environmental responsibility.

Restorative justice is another practice that reflects the principles of holistic governance. Instead of prioritizing severe and repressive punishments, this approach proposes the resolution of conflicts through dialogue, reconciliation, and reparation of the damages caused. Applied in various areas, from judicial systems to mediation of community conflicts, restorative justice promotes social cohesion and strengthens ties of solidarity.

Technology and innovation play an essential role in holistic governance. The use of artificial intelligence, data analysis, and digital platforms can improve governmental transparency and expand citizen participation. Systems for monitoring public policies, complaint applications, and online participation tools allow citizens to monitor and influence political decisions in real time. However, it is fundamental that technology be developed and used in an ethical and responsible manner, ensuring that its benefits are accessible to all and that its social and environmental impacts are carefully considered.

Despite the advances, the implementation of holistic politics and governance faces significant challenges. Resistance to change, consolidated political and economic interests, and the complexity of governmental systems can hinder the transition to this model. The lack of resources and training for public managers also represents an obstacle, making essential the investment in political education and development of leaders committed to this vision.

However, the opportunities to expand this model are innumerable. The growth of global awareness about sustainability and social justice drives the demand for more inclusive and responsible policies. Furthermore, globalization and technology facilitate the exchange of knowledge and experiences between countries, allowing good practices to be adapted and replicated in different contexts.

Finally, the role of the citizen is indispensable for the construction of an effective holistic governance. In addition to voting and demanding transparency from rulers, each individual can contribute actively by engaging in community initiatives, promoting constructive dialogues, and adopting sustainable habits in their daily lives. Education and awareness are powerful tools to drive a cultural change towards a more just, balanced, and sustainable society.

By integrating these principles and practices, holistic politics and governance offer a promising path to face the challenges of the 21st century. The interconnection between different areas of society demands solutions that transcend fragmented and short-term approaches. By strengthening democratic participation, guaranteeing equity, and prioritizing sustainability, it is possible to create a governance model that promotes shared prosperity and a more harmonious future for all.

The construction of this new governance paradigm demands a continuous commitment to political innovation and cultural transformation. As more societies realize the ineffectiveness of traditional fragmented models, the need to invest in leaders capable of articulating systemic and inclusive solutions grows. Political education, in this context, plays an essential role, preparing citizens and managers to understand the complexity of contemporary challenges and collaborate in the formulation of public policies that really meet collective needs. This transition will not occur instantaneously, but each step towards a more holistic governance represents a significant advance in the construction of a more just and sustainable world.

In addition to structural changes, the adoption of holistic politics also requires a new look at the values that guide life in society. Exacerbated individualism and the prioritization of profit over collective well-being need to give way to principles based on cooperation, ethics, and co-responsibility. Models that value transparency and the active participation of the population demonstrate that it is possible to balance economic development with social justice and environmental preservation. The challenge lies in transforming these ideas into concrete and lasting actions, resisting the pressures of those who profit from maintaining the status quo.

Holistic governance is not just a theoretical concept, but an urgent necessity in a world that faces increasingly interconnected challenges. As new experiences show their positive results, it becomes evident that fragmented solutions are no longer sufficient. The future depends on the collective capacity to rethink politics as a tool for real transformation, capable of building more resilient, balanced, and prosperous societies. By adopting a systemic, collaborative, and sustainable vision,

In addition to structural changes, the adoption of holistic politics also requires a new perspective on the values that guide life in society. Exacerbated individualism and the prioritization of profit over collective well-being need to give way to principles based on cooperation, ethics, and co-responsibility. Models that value transparency and the active participation of the population demonstrate that it is possible to balance economic development with social justice and environmental preservation. The challenge lies in transforming these ideas into concrete and lasting actions, resisting the pressures of those who profit from maintaining the status quo.

Holistic governance is not just a theoretical concept, but an urgent necessity in a world that faces increasingly interconnected challenges. As new experiences show their positive results, it becomes evident that fragmented solutions are no longer sufficient. The future depends on the collective capacity to rethink politics as a tool for real transformation, capable of building more resilient, balanced, and prosperous societies. By adopting a systemic, collaborative, and sustainable vision, humanity will be able to follow a path that transcends crises and establishes solid foundations for a better world.

Chapter 18
Ferramentas para a Integração

The rapid evolution of technology and innovation has profoundly redefined the way we live, work, and interact with the world. While these transformations bring significant advances in quality of life and efficiency of production processes, they also pose ethical, social, and environmental challenges that need to be carefully considered. Technological progress cannot be guided solely by the desire for growth and profit, but must be aligned with principles of equity, sustainability, and collective well-being. Adopting a holistic approach to technology and innovation requires consideration not only of immediate benefits but also of the long-term impacts on society, the environment, and future generations. This new paradigm seeks to integrate different fields of knowledge and promote solutions that respect the limits of the planet while expanding opportunities and social inclusion.

Technology has enormous potential to promote integration between individuals, communities, and nations, facilitating the exchange of knowledge and strengthening global collaboration networks. Advances in digital communications, artificial intelligence, and the internet of things have enabled the creation of new forms of interaction and cooperation, shortening distances and making information accessible to a growing number of people. However, unequal access to technology remains a significant obstacle, widening the digital divide and deepening social and economic inequalities. Truly holistic innovation must prioritize democratizing access to technological tools, ensuring that everyone can benefit from their advances and that no community is left behind by this progress. Furthermore, it is fundamental to promote digital literacy and critical thinking so that people can use technology consciously and responsibly, avoiding risks such as disinformation, data manipulation, and loss of privacy.

Innovation focused on sustainability is another essential pillar of this approach, as it allows us to face global challenges such as climate change, the depletion of natural resources, and environmental degradation. Emerging technologies, such as renewable energies, regenerative agriculture, biomaterials, and nature-based solutions, demonstrate that development can be compatible with environmental preservation and ecosystem regeneration. However, for these solutions to be widely adopted, a joint effort is needed between governments, companies, and civil society, promoting public policies that encourage sustainable production models and ensuring that innovation meets the needs of the present without compromising the possibilities of the future. True technological advancement lies not only in the creation of new products and services but also in the ability to shape a fairer, more balanced world prepared for the challenges ahead.

Technology has the power to connect people, ideas, and resources in ways previously unimaginable. The advancement of digital platforms, social networks, and communication tools has enabled individuals and communities to come together virtually to exchange knowledge, develop projects, and solve collective challenges. This connectivity has expanded opportunities for social, cultural, and economic integration, eliminating physical barriers and allowing dialogue between different realities. Today, companies can operate globally, professionals can collaborate regardless of their location, and social movements can gain strength rapidly through digital networks. This revolution in how we interact has brought immense potential for building a more interconnected and inclusive world.

However, despite all these advances, technology also has the power to create divisions. The digital divide is still a reality for millions of people who do not have access to devices, the internet, or sufficient technical knowledge to take advantage of the benefits of connectivity. In many places, digital infrastructure is still precarious or non-existent, perpetuating socioeconomic inequalities. In addition, the growth of information bubbles and the dissemination of polarizing content have contributed to social fragmentation and the reinforcement of prejudices and disinformation. Faced with these challenges, it is essential that technology be developed and used with a holistic approach, ensuring that its positive impact reaches all strata of society. The promotion of digital inclusion, through facilitated access to the internet, technological education, and public policies aimed at democratizing knowledge, is a fundamental step to ensure that no one is left behind by this progress.

Innovation, in addition to promoting connectivity, also plays a central role in the search for sustainable solutions. Faced with the environmental challenges that humanity faces, technological development must be aligned with principles of regeneration and preservation. Emerging technologies have shown that economic growth can go hand in hand with sustainability. Renewable energies, such as solar and wind, have become more accessible and efficient, allowing a transition to less polluting energy matrices. Precision agriculture, which uses sensors and artificial intelligence to optimize the use of inputs, reduces waste and the environmental impact of food production. Circular economy models propose the reuse and recycling of materials, reducing the extraction of natural resources and the accumulation of waste.

But for these innovations to be truly effective, it is necessary to integrate different perspectives and disciplines in the search for balanced solutions. A clear example of this are smart and sustainable cities, which combine various technologies to improve the quality of life of the population and increase urban resilience. The implementation of efficient and sustainable public transport systems, smart water supply networks, advanced waste management, and clean energy sources are essential steps to make urban centers more habitable and sustainable. However, for these solutions to be widely adopted, a joint effort is needed between governments, companies, and civil society, ensuring that innovations are accessible and beneficial to all.

In addition to connecting and driving sustainability, technology has also been a powerful ally in promoting well-being. Applications focused on mental and physical health, online learning platforms, virtual assistants for meditation, and physical activity monitoring programs are some examples of how technological advancement can contribute to improving quality of life. Today, an individual can access therapy online, learn a new language self-taught, or monitor their sleep habits with the help of smart devices. These resources increase people's autonomy over their own health and personal development.

However, the unrestrained use of technology can bring negative impacts, especially when there is no balance between the digital world and real life. The excess time spent on screens, the information overload, and the constant connection can lead to stress, anxiety, and social isolation. Dependence on digital devices can compromise sleep quality, interpersonal relationships, and even productivity at work. Therefore, it is fundamental to promote conscious use of technology, encouraging breaks, periods of disconnection, and face-to-face interactions. The balance between digital life and physical reality should be encouraged both in corporate environments and in educational and family contexts, so that the technological benefits are not obscured by their adverse effects.

Innovation and technology also raise ethical and social issues that cannot be ignored. The advancement of artificial intelligence and automation has brought profound impacts on the labor market, replacing some human functions with more efficient systems. While some sectors benefit from increased productivity, others face the reduction of jobs and the increase of social inequalities. In addition, user privacy is constantly threatened by the improper use of personal data, mass surveillance, and the manipulation of information. Companies and governments need to establish clear regulations to protect citizens and ensure that technological development is guided by ethics and transparency.

A holistic approach to technology requires that all these concerns be taken into account and that solutions be implemented to mitigate their risks. The creation of policies that regulate the use of data, the protection of digital rights, and the implementation of ethical guidelines in the development of artificial intelligence are fundamental measures. Furthermore, the active participation of society in decisions involving innovation and technology is essential to ensure that the solutions adopted are fair and representative.

Given the global scale of the challenges and opportunities that technology provides, collaboration between nations, organizations, and sectors becomes indispensable. The United Nations 2030 Agenda and the Sustainable Development Goals (SDGs) are examples of initiatives that encourage international cooperation for sustainable development. Partnerships between governments, private companies, universities, and non-governmental organizations enable the exchange of knowledge and the creation of joint solutions that benefit all of humanity. Citizen science, in which individuals contribute to research and data analysis, demonstrates how popular participation can strengthen innovation and generate positive impacts on a large scale.

Although the role of large institutions is fundamental, each individual can also contribute to a more responsible and sustainable use of technology. Small changes in daily life, such as reducing the consumption of unnecessary electronic devices, supporting sustainable innovation projects, and practicing a balanced use of technology, can generate important cumulative impacts. Awareness of the impacts of innovation and the adoption of habits that prioritize collective well-being are essential steps towards building a more integrated and harmonious future.

In a world where technology evolves rapidly and redefines our way of living, thinking, and interacting, it is fundamental to ensure that this evolution is guided by values that promote equity, sustainability, and social well-being. Adopting a holistic approach means not only maximizing technological benefits but also minimizing their risks and ensuring that their advantages are accessible to all. With collaboration between individuals, companies, governments, and organizations, we can create a future where innovation not only solves problems but also inspires a fairer, more balanced world prepared for the challenges of tomorrow.

The transition to a truly integrated society depends on how we choose to use technological tools in our favor. Progress is not defined only by the sophistication of innovations but by the positive impact they generate on people's lives and on the preservation of the planet. The search for inclusive and sustainable solutions requires a critical look at the consequences of digital advancement, ensuring that it serves to strengthen social bonds, reduce inequalities, and promote balanced development. The challenge, therefore, lies not only in the creation of new technologies but in the construction of a culture that values their ethical and responsible application.

Furthermore, continuous collaboration between different sectors will be essential to shape this new scenario. Governments need to create regulations that encourage the conscious use of innovation, while companies must incorporate environmental and social commitments into their strategies. Academia and civil society also play fundamental roles, broadening the debate on the impacts of technology and encouraging the active participation of citizens in defining guidelines for its development. Only through a joint effort will it be possible to ensure that technological advancement becomes an engine of inclusion and sustainability, rather than a factor of exclusion and degradation.

The path to a more integrated and balanced future lies in how we use the available resources to create a lasting positive impact. Technology, when combined with principles of equity and regeneration, can be a powerful tool to transform reality and prepare the next generations for increasingly complex challenges. It is up to each of us, as individuals and as a collectivity, to decide whether we want to be mere consumers of innovations or active agents in the construction of a world where technology is synonymous with connection, harmony, and shared prosperity.

Chapter 19
Celebrating Unity in Plurality

Cultural diversity is one of humanity's greatest riches, reflecting the complexity and depth of the human experience throughout history. Each culture carries a unique set of values, beliefs, traditions, and artistic expressions that shape individual and collective identities. However, in an increasingly globalized world, there is a growing risk that this diversity will be erased by cultural homogenization, where local practices and customs are replaced by dominant patterns. To avoid this invaluable loss, it is essential to adopt an approach that recognizes and celebrates plurality, promoting mutual respect and harmonious integration between different traditions.

Valuing diversity does not mean simply preserving the past but also creating spaces where different cultures can coexist, positively influence each other, and evolve together. By viewing culture as a dynamic field of exchange and learning, we can build richer, more resilient, and more inclusive societies in which the identity of each group is respected without implying isolation or conflict.

Cultural plurality, when recognized and encouraged, strengthens the social fabric, making communities more adaptable to changes and better prepared to face global challenges. In times of crisis, the diversity of perspectives and solutions offered by different traditions can be a decisive factor for innovation and overcoming difficulties. However, building a truly pluralistic society requires more than simply accepting differences; it requires the active promotion of intercultural dialogue and inclusion.

This means creating opportunities for all voices to be heard, ensuring that historically marginalized cultures have space to express themselves and contribute to social development. Education has a crucial role in this process, as by teaching about different cultures and traditions, it helps combat prejudices and stereotypes, promoting a broader and more empathetic view of the world. Furthermore, public policies and private initiatives can play an important role in protecting cultural heritage and valuing diversity in all aspects of social, economic, and political life.

Technology and media play an ambiguous role in this dynamic: while they can be used to broaden the visibility of diverse cultures and foster global exchange, they can also reinforce inequalities and promote a standardized view of cultural identity. Social networks, streaming platforms, and other digital tools offer unprecedented reach for cultural groups to share their artistic expressions and narratives, allowing traditions previously restricted to a local context to be appreciated globally. However, this democratization of access to culture must be accompanied by a conscious effort to ensure that all representations are authentic and respectful, avoiding cultural appropriation and the distortion of meanings.

The contemporary challenge is not only to preserve cultural diversity but also to ensure that this diversity can manifest itself in a fair and balanced way in an interconnected world. Celebrating unity in plurality means recognizing that, although we have distinct origins, histories, and customs, we are all interconnected by a common humanity, and it is this interconnection that allows us to build a richer, more harmonious, and sustainable future.

Cultural diversity presents itself as a vivid expression of human creativity and adaptability, reflecting the countless ways in which peoples, throughout history, have shaped their identities, beliefs, and traditions. Each culture carries its own legacy, a baggage of values and practices that enrich not only those who are part of it but all of humanity. The coexistence of these multiple perspectives offers the opportunity for constant learning, broadening horizons, and providing innovative solutions to common challenges. By observing cultural exchange, we see how different societies have found unique ways of dealing with nature, spirituality, interpersonal relationships, and technological advances. It is in this mosaic of experiences that the true richness of diversity resides: it allows us to learn from each other, to explore new paths, and to build bridges between different ways of seeing and being in the world.

More than a source of learning, cultural diversity also represents a pillar of resilience for societies. In times of crisis, be they environmental, economic, or social, the diversity of approaches and solutions provided by different traditions can be crucial to overcoming difficulties. When a community values its plurality, it becomes more flexible, able to reinvent itself and find alternatives to unexpected challenges. In contrast, societies that neglect their diversity or that impose forced uniformity tend to lose part of their vitality, becoming less prepared to face abrupt changes. Thus, the preservation of cultural diversity is not only a matter of respect for traditions but also an essential strategy for sustainability and collective well-being.

However, this richness faces constant challenges, especially in a world where globalization can, simultaneously, broaden access to different cultures and promote the homogenization of customs. The advancement of communications and large cultural industries often results in the predominance of certain cultural expressions to the detriment of others, leading to the marginalization of local traditions and the gradual loss of identities. Indigenous peoples, traditional communities, and minority ethnic groups often see their languages disappear, their customs ignored, and their lands threatened. Furthermore, cultural diversity can, in some situations, be a source of tension, especially when different groups compete for space, resources, or recognition. Prejudice and discrimination arise when difference is seen as an obstacle, rather than a meeting point. To overcome these challenges, it is essential to adopt an approach that promotes dialogue, mutual respect, and cooperation between different groups, ensuring that all cultures have space to express themselves and develop.

It is in this context that the concept of unity in plurality arises, an idea that recognizes diversity as an enriching force while seeking to promote harmony and collaboration between different cultures. This vision does not ignore differences; on the contrary, it celebrates them as fundamental elements of the human experience. However, it emphasizes that, despite distinct origins and histories, there is something essential that connects all human beings: the capacity to share, learn, and build together. Unity in plurality does not mean uniformity but rather the creation of an environment where different traditions can coexist respectfully and productively. This implies concrete efforts to value diversity, such as the promotion of intercultural dialogue, the valorization of cultural expressions, and the creation of spaces where multiple identities can flourish without fear of exclusion or repression.

To celebrate cultural diversity in a meaningful way, it is necessary to adopt practices and initiatives that reinforce respect, inclusion, and mutual understanding. One of the main paths to this is intercultural education, which seeks to teach not only the history and traditions of different peoples but also to encourage the exchange of experiences between individuals from diverse backgrounds. Schools and universities play a crucial role by incorporating content that promotes awareness of cultural plurality and combats stereotypes. In addition, festivals and cultural celebrations represent powerful tools for integration, providing opportunities for people to experience new forms of art, music, cuisine, and customs, thereby promoting the valorization and acceptance of differences.

The implementation of public policies focused on inclusion and diversity is also essential to ensure that all cultures have voice and visibility in different spheres of society. This includes measures such as representativeness in the media, equal opportunities in the labor market, and incentives for local cultural production. Intercultural dialogue should be encouraged both at the community level and in large international forums, creating spaces for different peoples to share their worldviews and strengthen ties of cooperation. At the same time, the preservation of cultural heritage should be a priority, ensuring that monuments, languages, rituals, and ancestral knowledge are protected and transmitted to future generations. Museums, libraries, and cultural centers play a vital role in this process, functioning as guardians of humanity's collective memory.

Technology and media, in turn, assume an ambiguous position in this scenario. If, on the one hand, they offer an unprecedented platform for the dissemination of cultures and narratives previously restricted to small groups, on the other, they can also reinforce stereotypes and promote a distorted view of diversity. Access to the internet allows artists, writers, and communities to share their cultural expressions with a global audience, democratizing cultural production and consumption. However, this same virtual space can be dominated by large conglomerates that standardize content and impose certain cultural trends on a worldwide scale. To ensure that technology is an ally in valuing diversity, it is essential that it be used ethically and responsibly, encouraging the plurality of voices and ensuring that all cultural representations are made authentically and respectfully.

Despite the challenges that the promotion of cultural diversity faces, there are countless opportunities to broaden its recognition and appreciation. The growing awareness of the importance of inclusion has led governments, businesses, and organizations to adopt more sensitive policies to diversity. In addition, globalization, when well directed, can facilitate cultural exchange and encourage collaboration between different peoples. The emergence of international cooperation networks, the strengthening of social movements, and the growth of digital activism are indicative that there is a global movement in favor of diversity and cultural justice.

In the end, culture and diversity are expressions of the richness and complexity of the human experience. By embracing unity in plurality, we not only promote respect and inclusion but also build a more harmonious, sustainable, and interconnected world. Cultural diversity teaches us that, regardless of differences, there are always points of convergence capable of uniting us. When we recognize and value this plurality, we create a future where all voices are heard, all stories are told, and all cultures are celebrated.

The construction of a world that celebrates unity in plurality requires a continuous commitment to empathy and mutual respect. In a global scenario where cultural boundaries become increasingly fluid, it is fundamental that societies encourage spaces for exchange and learning, ensuring that each culture can maintain its identity without fear of erasure or domination. This implies not only recognizing the importance of traditions but also creating opportunities for different groups to collaborate and contribute to a shared future. The true richness of diversity lies not only in its existence but in the way it is experienced and valued in everyday life.

However, this path is not without challenges. Intercultural dialogue needs to overcome historical barriers of prejudice, inequality, and exclusion, often reinforced by social and economic structures that privilege certain narratives at the expense of others. For plurality to be a force of cohesion and not fragmentation, it is essential that public policies, educational initiatives, and cultural productions work actively to dismantle stereotypes and build a society where all voices have space. Cultural plurality should not only be tolerated but celebrated and encouraged as a pillar of harmonious coexistence and sustainable development.

In the end, unity in plurality reminds us that, despite our differences, we share a common essence: the ability to create, evolve, and connect with one another. When we learn to see diversity as an opportunity for mutual enrichment, we broaden our understanding of the world and strengthen the bonds that unite us as humanity. The challenge is ongoing, but the reward is immeasurable: a future where all cultures can flourish together, building a more just, vibrant, and resilient society.

Chapter 20
Building an Inclusive World

The pursuit of social justice and equity is one of the fundamental cornerstones for building more harmonious, sustainable, and prosperous societies. In a world marked by structural inequalities and historical exclusions, ensuring that all people have access to equal opportunities and rights is not only a moral issue but also an essential requirement for human and social development. Equity goes beyond mere formal equality; it recognizes that different groups face distinct barriers and, therefore, requires the implementation of policies and practices that correct these disparities, ensuring that everyone can reach their full potential. Social justice, in turn, is not limited to the distribution of resources but involves creating conditions that allow the active and dignified participation of all citizens in economic, political, and cultural life. Only when these principles are incorporated into institutional structures and daily practices does it become possible to build truly inclusive societies, where no one is left behind.

For social justice and equity to be effectively promoted, it is fundamental to address inequalities in all their dimensions – economic, social, racial, gender, and environmental. Access to quality education, health, dignified work, and housing are basic rights that must be guaranteed to all, regardless of origin or socioeconomic condition. However, in many parts of the world, these rights are still privileges restricted to certain groups, perpetuating cycles of exclusion and vulnerability. The adoption of affirmative action policies and social protection mechanisms is essential to break this pattern and create an environment where every individual has the opportunity to contribute to society in a meaningful way. Furthermore, social justice must also consider the relationship between human beings and the environment, ensuring that natural resources are preserved and distributed fairly, respecting the needs of future generations. In this way, equity and sustainability become inseparable concepts, as a socially just world can only be built on solid ecological foundations.

Technology and innovation play a crucial role in promoting social justice and equity, provided they are used ethically and inclusively. Digital tools can democratize access to information, expand educational opportunities, and facilitate citizen participation in political and social processes. However, the technological revolution can also deepen inequalities if its access is restricted to certain groups or if it is used to reinforce systems of surveillance and control. Therefore, it is essential to ensure that innovation is guided by values of transparency, responsibility, and inclusion, promoting solutions that benefit the whole of society. In addition to institutional policies, the role of the individual is also fundamental in this process. Small actions, such as supporting local initiatives, combating prejudices, engaging in community projects, and raising awareness about social issues, contribute to the construction of a culture of equity and respect. By understanding social justice as a collective and continuous commitment, it is possible to transform existing structures and create a future where the dignity and rights of all are fully recognized and protected.

Social justice and equity are grounded in essential principles that guide the construction of a fairer and more inclusive society. The first of these is equality of opportunities, which ensures that all people, regardless of their origin, socioeconomic condition, race, gender, or any other characteristic, have unrestricted access to quality education, health services, employment opportunities, and political participation. This principle recognizes that, although people are different, none of them should be prevented from reaching their full potential due to structural barriers.

Another essential principle is respect for human dignity. Every individual has intrinsic value and must be treated with respect and consideration, regardless of their social position or condition. This implies the protection of fundamental human rights and the fight against any form of discrimination, ensuring that all voices are heard and respected in society.

Inclusion and participation are also fundamental pillars. It is not enough for rights to be formally guaranteed; it is necessary to ensure that all people can fully exercise their citizenship, actively participating in social, economic, and political life. This means creating accessible, representative, and welcoming spaces for historically marginalized groups, ensuring that their presence and contribution are valued.

In addition, social justice seeks to reduce inequalities in all their forms – social, economic, and environmental. For this, policies are needed that promote the fair redistribution of resources and opportunities, correcting distortions that perpetuate exclusion and vulnerability. This principle recognizes that equity does not mean treating everyone the same way, but rather offering differentiated support to ensure that everyone has real conditions for development and well-being.

Finally, social justice needs to be aligned with sustainability and intergenerational equity. The commitment to a fairer world should not be restricted to the needs of the present but should also consider the impact of actions on future generations. This requires sustainable development that respects environmental limits, preserves natural resources, and ensures that future generations inherit a habitable and balanced planet.

However, the implementation of these principles faces considerable challenges. Discrimination, poverty, social exclusion, and unequal access to resources and opportunities are persistent obstacles that are interconnected and reinforce each other, perpetuating cycles of marginalization. Globalization and rapid technological changes, if not accompanied by inclusive policies, can further accentuate these disparities, concentrating wealth and power in a few groups and leaving others on the margins.

To address these challenges, it is necessary to adopt a holistic approach, considering the interdependence of social, economic, and environmental systems. This means recognizing that social justice cannot be achieved in isolation but requires the articulation of diverse policies and initiatives that operate in an integrated and coordinated manner.

Among the strategies to promote social justice and equity, inclusion and affirmative action policies stand out. These measures seek to correct structural inequalities, ensuring that historically excluded groups have access to opportunities and resources. Examples of this include quotas in universities and in the labor market, training programs for vulnerable populations, and incentives for small entrepreneurs from marginalized communities. These actions not only offer immediate support but also contribute to the construction of a more representative and equitable society.

Education for citizenship and human rights is another powerful tool in this process. By promoting knowledge about rights and duties, stimulating critical thinking, and encouraging civic engagement, this approach contributes to the formation of more conscious and active citizens in the struggle for a fairer society. Schools, universities, and social organizations play a fundamental role in this sense, providing spaces for learning and reflection on themes such as diversity, equity, and democratic participation.

Universal access to health and education is also essential to reduce inequalities and guarantee dignity to all. Strong and well-structured public systems allow the entire population to have access to quality services, regardless of their income. This includes the expansion of hospitals and care units, the valorization of health professionals, and the implementation of educational programs that guarantee meaningful learning from childhood to adulthood.

In addition, the promotion of employment and decent work is one of the pillars of social justice. This involves not only the generation of jobs but also the guarantee of decent conditions for workers. Fair wages, safety in the workplace, respect for labor rights, and opportunities for professional growth are essential factors to ensure that all people can have a dignified and productive life.

Another crucial aspect is social protection and poverty reduction. For this, the implementation of social safety nets that support the most vulnerable in moments of crisis is fundamental. Income transfer programs, unemployment insurance, pensions, and access to basic services are mechanisms that prevent individuals and families from falling into extreme poverty, guaranteeing a minimum of dignity and stability.

Technology and innovation also play a significant role in promoting social justice, provided they are used in an ethical and inclusive manner. Digital tools can facilitate access to information, expand educational opportunities, and enable new forms of political and social participation. However, if access to these technologies is unequal or if they are used to reinforce mechanisms of surveillance and control, they can further deepen existing disparities. Therefore, it is essential that technological development is guided by principles of transparency, responsibility, and inclusion.

The promotion of social justice and equity, however, is not exempt from challenges. Resistance to change, lack of resources, and the complexity of social and economic systems can hinder the implementation of effective policies. Even so, there are also many opportunities. The growing awareness of the importance of equity is driving global movements and initiatives that demand structural transformations. In addition, new technologies and globalization, when well directed, can open paths for greater collaboration and exchange of ideas, facilitating the construction of fairer and more egalitarian societies.

Although governments, businesses, and organizations play a crucial role in this process, individuals can also contribute significantly. Small daily attitudes can have an important cumulative impact in building a more inclusive culture. Supporting local businesses, participating in community initiatives, combating prejudices in everyday life, and raising awareness about social issues are accessible and concrete ways to contribute to a fairer world.

Education and awareness, in turn, are fundamental tools for a lasting cultural transformation. When people adopt values and practices that promote inclusion, respect, and solidarity, they create an environment conducive to structural change. Social justice and equity are not just goals to be achieved but continuous commitments that require active participation and collective engagement. Only in this way will it be possible to build a future where all people have equal opportunities and are treated with dignity and respect.

The construction of a truly inclusive world requires a collective and constant effort, which goes beyond good intentions and speeches. It is necessary to transform social, economic, and political structures to ensure that all people, regardless of their origin, have access to the same opportunities. This involves everything from the implementation of effective public policies to profound cultural changes that encourage empathy and recognition of human dignity. Inclusion does not mean only opening spaces but ensuring that all voices are heard, respected, and valued.

However, inclusion will only be fully achieved if it is accompanied by a continuous commitment to equity and social justice. This means combating systemic inequalities, correcting historical disparities, and ensuring that achievements are sustainable over time. Innovation and technology, when used responsibly, can be powerful allies in this process, expanding access to essential resources and promoting new forms of social engagement. But no tool will replace the need for a genuine human effort to transform societies from the inside out.

The future of an inclusive world depends on the choices made in the present. Every action that promotes respect, empathy and cooperation strengthens the foundations for a more just and balanced society. Diversity and equity are not just abstract ideals, but essential foundations for sustainable and collective progress. By recognizing the importance of inclusion in all spheres of life, we take an essential step towards building a world where all people can live with dignity, opportunity and belonging.

Chapter 21
Holistic Utopias and Dystopias

Conceptions of the future reflect both our deepest desires and our darkest fears. Since the dawn of civilization, humanity has projected ideal worlds where justice, prosperity, and balance prevail, while simultaneously worrying about scenarios of collapse, where inequality, environmental degradation, and oppression become predominant. The holistic view emerges as an essential approach to shaping these projections, offering an integrative path that recognizes the interdependence between society, the environment, and technology. By understanding the complexity of natural and human systems, holistic thinking allows us to chart strategies that harmonize innovation and tradition, progress and preservation, seeking a sustainable balance for future generations. Thus, it becomes possible to build societies that value collective well-being, social justice, and the preservation of ecosystems, minimizing the risks inherent in dystopian models and maximizing the transformative potential of utopias.

The holistic perspective, unlike fragmented approaches, proposes an expanded vision of the future, in which all aspects of human existence are interconnected. Instead of just imagining technologically advanced societies or environmentally sustainable communities in isolation, this approach emphasizes the need for integration between scientific innovation, ancestral wisdom, and equitable social practices. This implies rethinking economic structures, educational models, and forms of political organization so that they promote both individual development and collective well-being. Technology, for example, can be a powerful ally in building a sustainable future, as long as it is used ethically and responsibly, avoiding its instrumentalization for social control or unbridled exploitation of resources. Similarly, strengthening community values and reconnecting with nature are fundamental to mitigating the negative impacts of modernity and fostering a more harmonious and resilient world.

By projecting future scenarios from this integrative perspective, it becomes clear that the construction of a holistic utopia does not depend only on technological advances or innovative public policies, but also on a profound transformation in the way we perceive and relate to the world. This requires a collective awakening to the importance of empathy, cooperation, and shared responsibility, recognizing that each individual choice influences the balance of the whole. If dystopias emerge from the disconnection between the fundamental elements of life—be they social, environmental, or spiritual—then the solution to avoid them lies precisely in valuing interdependence and commitment to a more just and sustainable future. In this way, instead of fearing what is to come, it is possible to take an active stance in building a tomorrow that reflects the principles of harmony, equity, and shared prosperity.

The concept of the future has always oscillated between utopian aspirations and dystopian fears, reflecting the hopes and anxieties of humanity. The holistic vision emerges as an essential approach to shaping these projections, seeking to integrate society, the environment, and technology in a sustainable balance. This perspective is not limited to technological advances or innovative public policies but proposes a profound transformation in the way we perceive and relate to the world. Thus, it is necessary to recognize the interdependence of systems and adopt an active commitment to a future that values harmony, equity, and shared prosperity.

Holistic utopia, as the ultimate expression of this ideal, presents a scenario where human well-being, environmental sustainability, and social justice coexist in balance. This idealized future is built on fundamental pillars that guarantee the integrity of natural and social systems, promoting harmonious and sustainable coexistence. The first of these pillars is ecological sustainability, in which society operates in synergy with nature. Resources are used regeneratively, ensuring that future generations do not inherit a degraded world. Cities are designed to be green, resilient, and efficient spaces, with energy systems based on renewable sources and accessible and ecological public transport. Bioclimatic architecture, urban reforestation, and regenerative agriculture become essential practices, allowing urban environments to integrate organically with ecosystems.

Another fundamental aspect of holistic utopia is social justice and equity, ensuring that all individuals have access to the essential resources for a dignified life. Education is universal and inclusive, promoting not only technical knowledge but also emotional and ethical intelligence. Health is treated holistically, considering not only the physical but also the mental and spiritual aspects. The economy is structured cooperatively, reducing inequalities and strengthening local communities. Models of universal basic income, solidarity economy, and complementary social currencies are adopted to ensure that no one is left on the margins of society.

Furthermore, integral well-being is a central principle of this idealized society. Holistic medicine, combined with modern science, proposes treatments that consider the human being in their totality, balancing body and mind. Practices such as meditation, yoga, and natural therapies are incorporated into everyday life, strengthening the connection between individuals and promoting a more harmonious life. Emotional balance is valued as much as physical health, ensuring that interpersonal relationships are based on respect and empathy.

Technology plays a crucial role but is developed and applied responsibly. Artificial intelligence, robotics, and biotechnology are directed to solve global challenges such as combating hunger, curing diseases, and mitigating climate change. Instead of fostering inequalities or being used as a tool of control, technology serves the common good, being regulated by rigorous ethical principles and popular participation.

Culture and diversity are celebrated in this utopia because valuing different traditions and forms of expression strengthens collective identity and promotes a more inclusive world. The exchange of knowledge between cultures and the preservation of ancestral knowledge are encouraged, creating a society that honors its past while building an innovative future.

On the other hand, the holistic dystopia represents the collapse of these principles, resulting in a world of inequality, environmental degradation, and disconnection. In this scenario, the unbridled exploitation of natural resources leads to the destruction of ecosystems, making the planet a hostile environment for life. Rampant pollution, water and food scarcity, and the disappearance of species create an unsustainable environment, where climate change spirals out of control and natural disasters become constant.

Social inequality reaches extreme levels, with a small elite monopolizing wealth and resources while the majority of the population lives in precarious conditions. Human rights are ignored, and social justice becomes non-existent. Authoritarian and repressive government systems emerge, exacerbating collective suffering. Technology, instead of liberating, becomes an instrument of surveillance and manipulation, eliminating privacy and free will. Artificial intelligence is used for population control, reinforcing the concentration of power and the exploitation of the working class, which finds itself replaced by automated systems without any support.

Social fragmentation intensifies in this dystopian reality. Emotional isolation and lack of empathy erode the foundations of human coexistence, leading to widespread conflict. Community ties are weakened, and people become increasingly alienated, trapped in information bubbles controlled by algorithms that reinforce divisions and intolerances. The sense of purpose and belonging dissolves, making existence an incessant search for fleeting pleasures and uncontrolled consumption.

Faced with these extreme possibilities, holistic thinking emerges as an essential tool for building a balanced future. It allows us to understand the interconnections between human and natural systems, facilitating the identification of paths that avoid dystopian scenarios and promote utopian visions. The systemic view makes it possible to anticipate impacts and create integrated solutions, while prevention and resilience become fundamental strategies for dealing with future challenges. Collaboration and dialogue between different sectors and cultures reinforce the idea that progress must be collective, ensuring that technological innovations are conducted ethically and responsibly.

Education plays a central role in this process, as awareness of the interdependence of systems promotes the adoption of more sustainable and just practices. Educational models focused on the integral development of the human being empower new generations to face complex challenges with creativity and empathy, shaping citizens aware of their role in society and the environment.

Despite the challenges inherent in building this desirable future—such as resistance to change, scarcity of resources, and the complexity of global systems—there are significant opportunities. The increasing collective awareness of the importance of sustainability and social justice drives the search for more holistic and integrated approaches. Technology and globalization, when used purposefully, facilitate the dissemination of innovative ideas and strengthen collaborative networks that can accelerate this transformation.

The future, after all, is not a predetermined destination but a continuous construction based on the choices and actions of humanity. By embracing a holistic perspective, we can guide these choices consciously, promoting societies that balance innovation and tradition, development and preservation, individuality and collectivity. In this way, instead of fearing the challenges of tomorrow, we can take an active role in creating a world that reflects the principles of harmony, equity, and shared prosperity.

The realization of a future based on holistic utopia, therefore, requires collective engagement and a profound change in the way we structure our social, economic, and environmental relations. This process does not occur abruptly or uniformly but through small progressive transformations, driven by local and global initiatives that demonstrate, in practice, the viability of this model. Projects for sustainable cities, economic systems based on cooperation, and educational policies aimed at the integral formation of the human being are examples of how this future can begin to materialize. The transition demands resilience and adaptation, but the commitment to this construction paves the way for a civilization that is more aware of its role in planetary balance.

Still, the challenges inherent in implementing this vision cannot be underestimated. The clash between political and economic interests, resistance to cultural changes, and the complexity of environmental crises require dynamic and adaptable solutions. The holistic approach does not seek unique or immutable answers, but rather the ability to see beyond the immediate, reconciling progress and sustainability in a flexible and innovative way. To prevent dystopias from becoming irreversible realities, it is essential to cultivate a long-term mentality that prioritizes the common good and encourages global cooperation. Commitment to this ideal is not just a matter of survival, but a testament to the human capacity to evolve and reimagine its own destiny.

Thus, the choice between holistic utopias and dystopias is not a mere exercise in futuristic speculation, but a shared responsibility, the consequences of which depend on decisions made in the present. The future is shaped not only by major scientific advances or structural changes but by the daily lives of each individual who, by recognizing their interconnection with the whole, begins to act in a more conscious and ethical way. It is in this space between action and vision that lies the true transformative potential of humanity, capable of building a tomorrow where harmony, justice, and sustainability are more than ideals, but the foundations of a new reality.

Chapter 22
Converging Towards a New Reality

The understanding of reality has always been at the heart of the human journey, driven by both scientific inquiry and spiritual experience. Science, with its empirical and rational method, has unveiled the mechanisms of the material universe, providing extraordinary advances in technology, medicine, and the understanding of nature. In parallel, spirituality has offered a deeper meaning to existence, exploring subjective and transcendent dimensions of life. Although often seen as opposites, these two approaches need not be mutually exclusive. On the contrary, they can converge to form a broader and more integrated view of the world, in which rational knowledge and intuitive wisdom complement each other. The search for the ultimate understanding of reality requires not only explanations about how the universe works, but also reflections on the meaning and purpose of human existence within this vast cosmic scenario.

This convergence between science and spirituality becomes increasingly evident as new discoveries challenge established paradigms. In quantum physics, for example, phenomena such as non-locality and entanglement suggest that the interconnectedness of the universe goes beyond what classical logic can explain. Similarly, studies in neuroscience demonstrate that spiritual practices, such as meditation and contemplation, cause significant changes in the structure and activity of the brain, improving mental and emotional health. Ecology, in turn, reinforces the idea that all life forms are interconnected, echoing ancient spiritual traditions that view the Earth as a living and sacred organism. These advances not only validate ancient spiritual perspectives, but also expand the very notion of reality within the scientific scope, revealing a complexity that transcends the limits of matter and direct observation.

By integrating science and spirituality, a path opens to a more complete and harmonious understanding of the universe and the position of the human being within it. This dialogue does not mean replacing one field with the other, but rather recognizing that both offer valuable contributions. Science provides tools to understand natural phenomena, develop technologies and improve the quality of life, while spirituality helps in building values, in the search for a purpose and in cultivating a sense of belonging to the cosmos. This synthesis allows not only intellectual and technological advances, but also a more balanced development of humanity, promoting a future where knowledge and wisdom go hand in hand.

The separation between science and spirituality has deep roots in Western history, especially in the Enlightenment, a period in which reason and empiricism were enshrined as the fundamental pillars of knowledge.

During this time, the search for truth became guided almost exclusively by the scientific method, which established itself as the legitimate way to understand reality. The accelerated advance of science and technology brought undeniable achievements, but, in this process, subjective and metaphysical aspects of existence were left aside, often seen as mere irrational or superstitious beliefs. Materialism and reductionism became dominant, relegating spirituality to a lower plane, as if it were something incompatible with legitimate knowledge.

However, this fragmented view of the world is not universal. In various cultures and philosophical traditions, science and spirituality have never been antagonistic. In Buddhism, for example, the investigation of mind and reality is conducted both by meditative experience and rational observation. Taoism, in turn, understands nature as a dynamic and interconnected flow, something that modern physics is beginning to recognize. Indigenous philosophies have also always seen the cosmos as a great living organism, in which each being has an essential connection to the whole. In these systems of thought, reason and intuition coexist, and the search for knowledge is comprehensive, contemplating both the tangible and the intangible.

In recent centuries, however, the barrier between spirituality and science has been gradually questioned, as new scientific discoveries reveal aspects of reality that dialogue with concepts long defended by spiritual traditions. Quantum physics, for example, demonstrates that the universe is not composed of separate and independent entities, but rather by a web of dynamic relationships. The phenomenon of quantum entanglement indicates that distant particles can be mysteriously connected, influencing each other instantaneously, something that challenges the traditional mechanistic view. This principle resonates with ancestral spiritual ideas, which have always maintained that the separation between beings is an illusion and that all existence is interconnected by invisible forces.

Neuroscience, in turn, has explored the effects of spiritual practices on the brain and discovered concrete evidence that meditation, prayer and other contemplative techniques promote significant structural and functional changes. Studies show that these practices increase the activity of brain areas associated with empathy, well-being and emotional regulation, while reducing the effects of stress and anxiety. This suggests that spirituality is not just a subjective or cultural construct, but something that has a measurable impact on human biology, reinforcing the idea that mind and body are not separate entities, but parts of an integrated system.

Modern ecology has also corroborated ancient spiritual views on the relationship between humans and nature. Research shows that ecosystems function as interdependent networks, where the balance of each element is essential for the maintenance of life. This perspective is reminiscent of the reverence for nature present in various spiritual traditions, which see it not as a set of resources to be exploited, but as a living and sacred entity. The concept of Gaia, which sees the Earth as a self-regulating organism, finds parallels in indigenous beliefs, which have always recognized the interdependence of all life forms.

Faced with this growing convergence between science and spirituality, a new approach to understanding reality emerges, which does not seek to replace one field with the other, but rather to integrate them in a complementary way. Science offers rigorous methods to investigate natural phenomena and develop technologies, while spirituality provides a broader perspective on the meaning and purpose of existence. This synthesis can bring significant benefits, allowing scientific advances to be guided by ethical principles and spirituality to rely on concrete evidence, strengthening its relevance in the contemporary world.

Spirituality can contribute to science in several ways. First, by offering a sense of meaning and purpose, it can help contextualize scientific discoveries within a broader view of existence. Science explains how things work, but often does not address why they exist or what their role is within a larger scenario. This gap can be filled by spirituality, which invites reflection on the value and purpose of life.

In addition, spirituality can serve as an ethical guide for scientific practice. Technological progress has brought enormous benefits, but also complex ethical challenges, such as the dilemmas of genetic engineering, artificial intelligence and the exploitation of natural resources. Spirituality, by emphasizing values such as compassion, responsibility and respect for life, can offer a moral compass to guide the use of scientific knowledge in a responsible and beneficial way for humanity.

Science, in turn, can enrich spirituality, providing empirical support for practices and beliefs that were once considered purely subjective. Studies on the effects of meditation, mindfulness and prayer show that these practices bring concrete benefits to physical and mental health, encouraging their integration into clinical and therapeutic contexts. In addition, research on consciousness raises fascinating questions about the nature of the "self" and its relationship to the universe, opening space for new interpretations on topics such as the continuity of consciousness after death, the interconnectedness of the mind and even mystical phenomena.

Science also has the power to awaken a deep sense of reverence for the universe. The vastness of the cosmos, the complexity of living organisms and the elegance of natural laws are sources of wonder and awe, something that many spiritual traditions have always emphasized. In this sense, science can inspire a spirituality based on wonder and contemplation of the beauty and mystery of existence.

However, this convergence between science and spirituality still faces challenges. Many scientists remain skeptical of any notion that seems to transcend the limits of materialism, while religious sectors may resist the incorporation of scientific concepts that contradict traditional interpretations. Reconciling these perspectives requires an open dialogue, based on mutual respect and a willingness to explore unknown territories without prejudice.

On the other hand, the opportunities for this encounter are immense. The world is increasingly interconnected, and the exchange of ideas between different cultures and disciplines has never been so accessible. This exchange allows the emergence of more holistic approaches, which combine the analytical rigor of science with the intuitive depth of spirituality. As humanity advances, the integration of these fields can lead us to a more complete understanding of reality, promoting a balance between reason and intuition, between knowledge and wisdom.

By uniting these two great forces of human thought, we can move towards a more integrated view of the universe and our place in it. This synthesis not only broadens the horizons of science and spirituality, but also inspires us to seek a more harmonious future, where knowledge is used responsibly and wisdom is cultivated as an essential pillar of life.

The convergence between science and spirituality, although still facing resistance, points to a new paradigm in which both reinforce each other. As science expands its horizons and questions boundaries previously considered insurmountable, it becomes evident that there are more layers to reality than classical materialism supposed. Similarly, spirituality finds a renewed space to express itself without needing to oppose rational thought, but rather by engaging with it in an enriching way. This complementarity allows the human being not only to better understand the world around him, but also to deepen his relationship with it, cultivating a more conscious and balanced existence.

This integration does not mean the disappearance of the distinctions between the two fields, but rather the recognition that both offer essential perspectives for the construction of a broader and more meaningful view of reality. Science, by revealing the complexity and interconnectedness of the universe, reinforces spiritual intuitions about the unity of existence, while spirituality can offer science an ethical and philosophical dimension that guides it towards a more responsible use of its advances. This encounter not only expands human knowledge, but also transforms the way we relate to knowledge itself, making it more inclusive, profound and aligned with the challenges of our time.

Thus, instead of an irreconcilable opposition, the convergence between science and spirituality can represent one of the most important evolutionary leaps of humanity. The future that emerges from this synthesis is one in which rational thought and intuition walk side by side, allowing the human being to explore not only the mysteries of the physical universe, but also those of consciousness and existence. On this path, the possibility of a new understanding opens up, where knowledge and wisdom unite to shape a more integrated, full and inspiring reality.

Chapter 23
Global Transformation

Global transformation does not occur in isolation or spontaneously; it is the result of a continuous process of changes that involve both large social structures and individual actions. In an interconnected world, where challenges such as the climate crisis, social inequalities, and technological advancement shape society, each person plays a fundamental role in building a more balanced and sustainable future. The impact of individual choices may seem small at first glance, but when added to the decisions of millions, it becomes a powerful force capable of redefining paradigms and driving significant change. Transformation begins at the personal level and expands to the collective, influencing political, economic, and environmental systems. Thus, every conscious action—from adopting more sustainable habits to engaging in social causes—contributes to a larger movement, where the sum of individual intentions translates into concrete impacts on global reality.

This transformation requires a new mindset, based on values such as empathy, collaboration, and respect for diversity. The competitive model that has prevailed for centuries, emphasizing individualism and the exploitation of resources without regard for long-term impacts, needs to give way to a more integrative and cooperative vision. The valuing of education, critical thinking, and social responsibility are essential pillars for this change. Access to knowledge allows people to understand the world's challenges and make informed decisions, whether in conscious consumption, political participation, or innovation in their fields of activity. In addition, technology and digital connectivity offer unprecedented opportunities for mobilization and exchange of ideas, allowing innovative solutions to be developed collaboratively and globally.

However, for this transformation to be effective, it is essential to overcome resistance and challenges that arise along the way. Structural changes often face opposition from vested interests, and ingrained habits can hinder the adoption of new practices. Still, history shows that societies evolve and adapt as new needs and values emerge. The strength of global transformation lies in the human capacity to reinvent itself, learn, and act collectively towards a greater purpose. Each individual who chooses to act with awareness and responsibility becomes a link in this chain of change, driving a more balanced and sustainable future for generations to come.

The individual is the basic unit of society and, as such, has the power to influence their surroundings in a meaningful way. Small changes in personal behavior can generate a significant cumulative impact, especially when adopted by millions of people around the world. Transformation begins with awareness, which allows the individual to understand global challenges and recognize their ability to contribute to change. Learning about issues such as climate change, social inequality, and biodiversity conservation is an essential first step. This education should not be passive; it must involve discussions, questioning, and the sharing of knowledge, expanding the network of impact.

In everyday life, small actions can make a big difference. Reducing excessive consumption, choosing sustainable products, and supporting local businesses are some ways to minimize environmental impact and strengthen fairer economies. Recycling and composting waste avoid the accumulation of garbage and help preserve natural resources. Opting for sustainable means of transport, such as bicycles, public transport or electric vehicles, significantly reduces the emission of polluting gases. In food, a more sustainable diet, based on conscious consumption and the appreciation of organic products, contributes both to personal health and to the preservation of the environment.

Civic engagement also plays a fundamental role in this process. Actively participating in political and social life, voting consciously, signing petitions, attending peaceful demonstrations, and supporting public policies aimed at social and environmental justice are ways of exercising citizenship. Structural change does not happen only at the individual level, but through collective pressure that leads governments and companies to adopt more responsible practices.

Furthermore, volunteering and social action are powerful ways to contribute directly to transformation.

Engaging in community projects, working with non-governmental organizations, and supporting local initiatives strengthens social bonds and provides positive impacts for vulnerable communities. Donations, mentoring, and social assistance programs help reduce inequalities and expand opportunities for those most in need.

Creativity and innovation also play a crucial role in building a more sustainable future. Each individual, within their abilities and talents, can develop innovative solutions to global challenges. Entrepreneurs can create socially responsible businesses, scientists can develop new sustainable technologies, and artists can use their art to inspire change and raise awareness in society. Human creative potential is a powerful tool to solve problems in innovative and effective ways.

Values and spirituality also have an essential role in this journey. Compassion and empathy allow people to connect with the difficulties of others and act in solidarity, promoting justice and inclusion. Respect for nature strengthens environmental awareness, encouraging practices that regenerate ecosystems and preserve biodiversity. The search for a life purpose aligned with the common good motivates actions aimed at a lasting positive impact.

Despite the challenges inherent in global transformation, such as resistance to change, lack of resources, and the complexity of social systems, there are increasing opportunities for individuals to contribute actively. The advancement of technology and globalization have facilitated the connection between people from different parts of the world, creating networks of support and collaboration that amplify the impact of individual actions. Social movements, digital initiatives, and awareness campaigns demonstrate how collective mobilization can generate significant change.

However, no transformation happens in isolation. The community plays an essential role as a space for multiplying individual actions into collective impacts. Support networks, such as cooperatives and community banks, strengthen the local economy and promote fairer and more sustainable consumption. The adoption of sustainable community practices, such as urban gardens, renewable energy, and recycling programs, helps build more resilient cities prepared for future challenges.

The active participation of the community in politics and decision-making is fundamental to strengthening participatory democracy. Popular assemblies, participatory budgeting, and community debates ensure that different voices are heard and that public policies reflect the real needs of the population.

Global transformation is a collective process that begins with the action of each individual. By integrating awareness, daily changes, civic engagement, and ethical values, each person contributes to a more just, sustainable, and harmonious future. The responsibility belongs to everyone, but it is also a unique opportunity to create a better world for future generations.

True global transformation is not just about structural and political changes, but about a revolution in collective consciousness. The way we see the world, others, and ourselves defines the directions we take as a society. The future will not be shaped only by innovative technologies or major reforms, but by the human capacity to cultivate empathy, cooperation, and a deep sense of responsibility for the planet and its inhabitants. When the understanding of interdependence becomes part of the global mindset, each action ceases to be isolated and becomes part of a continuous movement of regeneration and balance.

This process requires patience and perseverance, as true transformations rarely happen immediately. Each advance faces challenges, each new paradigm encounters resistance, but history shows that, over time, progressive and sustainable ideas consolidate and transform entire societies. What may seem like a small change in mindset today may, in the future, become the basis of a new world model. The commitment to this journey should not be based only on expectations of immediate results, but on the conviction that each step in the right direction is already, in itself, an achievement.

Global transformation, therefore, is not an isolated event, but a continuous process, driven by the sum of small and large actions over time. Every conscious choice, every sustainable innovation, every act of solidarity contributes to a more just and balanced world. If the future of humanity is uncertain, it is up to us to decide how we want to build it: with fear and inertia, or with courage and purpose. In the end, the change we seek for the world begins within each of us.

Chapter 24
The Search for the Meaning of Life

The search for the meaning of life is an intrinsic journey to the human experience, permeating all cultures, eras, and historical contexts. From the philosophers of antiquity to modern scientists, this question has been investigated from different perspectives, revealing that the meaning of existence is not a single and universal answer, but a personal and dynamic construction. For some, the meaning of life lies in the realization of aspirations and achievements; for others, in the connection with something greater, whether through spirituality, art, or human relationships. However, regardless of the approach taken, purpose and meaning arise when there is a harmonious integration between the physical, mental, emotional, and spiritual dimensions of existence. By considering this search holistically, one realizes that meaning is not isolated in a single aspect of life, but emerges from the interconnection between all experiences and the way each individual relates to themselves, to others, and to the universe around them.

Understanding this journey requires a deep dive into self-awareness and the recognition of external influences that shape our perception of purpose. Society, through cultural norms and expectations, often imposes definitions of what it means to have a meaningful life, associating it with professional success, the accumulation of material goods, or conformity to certain standards. However, true fulfillment is not limited to external goals, but to authenticity and the ability to align actions with deep inner values. Self-knowledge, therefore, becomes essential in this trajectory, allowing each person to explore their own interests, passions, and convictions to define a purpose that genuinely resonates with their essence. This process is not static, because as we evolve, our values and perceptions also transform, inviting us to constantly revisit what gives meaning to our existence.

Connection with the whole—whether with nature, with the collective, or with the transcendental aspect of life—represents one of the deepest paths to finding meaning. When one recognizes the interdependence between all things, a sense of belonging emerges that broadens the vision of individual purpose. Contributing to the well-being of the planet, cultivating relationships based on compassion, and developing a spirituality that promotes harmony are ways to expand this connection, enriching the life experience. In addition, moments of contemplation, meditation, and immersion in art or music can provide transcendent experiences that reinforce the feeling of integration with something greater. Thus, the search for the meaning of life is not just an abstract questioning, but a living process, built daily through choices, interactions, and reflections. By adopting a holistic approach, it is possible to understand that life does not need to have a single fixed meaning, but can be filled with multiple meanings, found in the richness of experiences and the depth of the connections we cultivate along the way.

The search for the meaning of life is a personal and unique journey, shaped by our experiences, values, beliefs, and the cultural context in which we are inserted. However, certain questions seem to be universal: why do we exist? What is the true purpose of life? How can we live meaningfully? These questions have accompanied humanity since the beginning and, although the answers may vary from individual to individual, there is a consensus that the meaning of life is not found isolated in a single dimension of existence, but rather in the integration of all of them. Holistic thinking suggests that it is necessary to consider the body, mind, emotions, and spirit as interconnected parts of a larger whole. In this way, this approach invites us to explore the totality of the human experience, seeking connections and meanings that transcend the isolated parts and are revealed at the intersection of all dimensions of being.

The search for the meaning of life unfolds in several dimensions, each contributing to the construction of a broader and deeper meaning. The physical dimension, for example, is the starting point for a balanced and full life. Caring for the body, through a healthy diet, regular exercise, and maintaining restful sleep, creates the essential foundation for us to explore other facets of existence. A healthy body gives us the disposition to experience experiences, provides us with energy to fulfill our aspirations, and keeps us connected to the material world in an active and present way.

The mental dimension involves the pursuit of knowledge and intellectual development. Continuous learning expands our understanding of the world and ourselves, providing tools to deal with life's challenges in a more conscious and reflective way. Education, reading, critical thinking, and the ability to question help us build our own meaning for existence, allowing us not to passively accept definitions imposed by society. Cultivating the mind is, therefore, a fundamental path to personal growth and the formulation of an authentic purpose.

The emotional dimension, in turn, invites us to delve into human relationships and the universe of emotions. Knowing how to manage our feelings, cultivating empathy, compassion, and love connects us more deeply with others, bringing a sense of belonging and purpose. Interpersonal relationships play a central role in constructing the meaning of life, because it is through them that we experience the joy of sharing, mutual support, and the satisfaction of contributing to the well-being of others. When we nurture genuine bonds and develop balanced emotional intelligence, we find clearer reasons to move forward, even in difficult times.

Finally, the spiritual dimension represents the search for connection with something greater than ourselves. This connection can manifest itself in different ways: for some, it occurs through religiosity and faith; for others, in the contemplation of nature, in the practice of meditation, or in immersion in existential questions. The spiritual aspect helps us to transcend the ego and realize that we are part of a larger reality, where everything is interconnected. Spirituality invites us to see life from a higher perspective, reframing pain, challenges, and achievements within a broader context of evolution and learning.

Within this journey, purpose emerges as a fundamental element. It gives us direction and motivation, making our actions and choices have a deeper meaning. However, contrary to what many imagine, purpose is not something fixed or external, which needs to be discovered as if it were a hidden secret. It is an ongoing construction that emerges from the interaction between our experiences and values. Finding purpose involves reflecting on our passions, talents, and how we can contribute to the world around us. For some, purpose can manifest itself in work; for others, in family, art, community service, or the incessant pursuit of knowledge. The important thing is to understand that it is dynamic, evolving throughout life as we grow and transform.

By understanding that we are interconnected with the whole, we broaden our vision of existence. Holistic thinking reminds us that we are not isolated beings, but part of an infinite network of relationships, which involves other people, nature, and even the universe. This connection can be a powerful source of meaning, bringing a sense of belonging that transcends individuality. There are several ways to strengthen this connection: contributing to the collective well-being, through community service and volunteering, is one of them. When we help others, we experience a deep sense of accomplishment, because we realize that our actions have a positive impact beyond ourselves.

Another way to connect with the whole is through reverence for nature. Observing the grandeur of the universe, contemplating the harmony of ecosystems, and recognizing the interdependence between all living beings awakens us to the importance of preserving and regenerating our planet. This sense of belonging to Earth inspires us to adopt sustainable practices, promoting a more respectful and balanced relationship with the environment.

In addition, transcendent experiences can broaden our perception of the meaning of life. Art, music, meditation, and contemplation of the cosmos are gateways to states of consciousness that make us feel part of something greater. These moments of deep connection help us break the ego barrier and see existence from a broader and more integrated perspective.

However, this journey in search of the meaning of life is not without its challenges. The complexity of existence, existential crises, and the pressure of modern society can hinder this search. Often, we are led to believe that the meaning of life must be associated with material success, productivity, or external recognition. However, overcoming these challenges involves developing a more authentic view of one's own life. Self-knowledge then becomes an essential tool. It allows us to understand our emotions, our values, and what truly motivates us, helping us to make decisions aligned with our true essence.

Resilience and the ability to adapt are also fundamental in this process. Life is constantly changing and, often, the meaning we give it needs to be revisited and reformulated as we face new experiences and challenges. Having the flexibility to adapt and find meaning even in difficult times allows us to grow and mature along the journey.

Another essential factor in overcoming the challenges of the search for meaning is connection with others. Having a support network, cultivating healthy relationships, and being inserted in supportive communities strengthens our sense of belonging and helps us to go through periods of uncertainty with more security and balance.

Within this context, spirituality also plays a crucial role. Whether through faith, philosophy, or contemplation of the mystery of existence, it invites us to seek a deeper understanding of who we are and our place in the universe. Often, it is in moments of crisis that we find meaningful answers and develop a clearer vision of our purpose and our connection to the whole.

The search for the meaning of life, therefore, is not a question with a single and definitive answer. On the contrary, it is a continuous process of discovery, growth, and transformation. By integrating the physical, mental, emotional, and spiritual dimensions, we are able to broaden our perception of the meaning of existence, finding purpose in the richness of the experiences we live and the connections we cultivate. Thus, embracing this journey with authenticity and openness allows us not only to discover our own meaning of life, but also to contribute to a more harmonious, just, and sustainable world.

The meaning of life, therefore, is not a fixed destination to be reached, but a path under constant construction, which is revealed in the experience of living fully. By accepting this journey as a dynamic process, we learn to deal with uncertainties without the need for absolute answers. True meaning emerges when we allow ourselves to explore, question, and grow, transforming each moment into an opportunity for learning and connection. The search for meaning does not have to be a distressing obsession, but an invitation to dive into existence with curiosity and openness, valuing both challenges and achievements.

Throughout this journey, the importance of the present becomes evident. Often, we are so concerned with finding a great purpose that we forget that the meaning of life is also found in small moments: in the exchange of glances with a loved one, in the pleasure of creating something new, in the feeling of belonging when admiring the vast starry sky. Life does not need to be defined only by great goals; it is also woven by simple gestures that make us feel alive and connected to the world around us. The purpose may lie in the way we love, how we share our joy, and how we contribute, however modestly, to the well-being of those around us.

Ultimately, finding meaning in life does not mean discovering a single universal truth, but building a meaning that resonates with who we are. Each one follows their own path, and there are no ready answers or definitive formulas. What there is, in reality, is the freedom to choose how we want to live, how we want to impact the world, and how we want to remember our own existence. When we face this search as a dance between reason and mystery, between the individual and the collective, we realize that the meaning of life is not an end to be achieved, but a story that unfolds every day, written by our experiences, choices, and connections.

Chapter 25
Living Holism in Daily Life

Living holistically means adopting a perspective that recognizes the interconnection between all spheres of existence, from individual well-being to collective and planetary balance. This approach is not limited to abstract concepts, but translates into daily choices and practices that promote harmony between body, mind, emotions, and spirit. In the modern world, where fragmentation and haste often distance people from their own essence, incorporating holism into daily life is an invitation to reclaim full consciousness, act with intention, and cultivate healthier relationships with oneself, with others, and with the surrounding environment. Small changes, when made consistently, have the power to create profound and sustainable transformations, extending individual impact to the community and global levels.

This experience begins with self-care and valuing the present experience. The body, as a vehicle for life's journey, needs to be nurtured and respected, whether through a balanced diet, adequate rest, or the practice of physical activities that promote vitality. On the mental plane, cultivating intellectual curiosity and critical reflection allows for a broader view of reality, avoiding reductionist views and stimulating creativity in solving challenges. In the emotional aspect, emotional intelligence becomes essential to develop relationships based on empathy, active listening, and mutual respect, strengthening bonds that sustain both personal growth and collective well-being. Spirituality, regardless of how it is expressed, offers a space for connection with something greater, providing meaning and purpose to daily actions. When all these dimensions are integrated, a more balanced flow of life is created, where each choice reflects a conscious commitment to one's own well-being and to the world.

Beyond personal development, living holistically means recognizing the impact of our actions on society and the planet. Choosing to consume consciously, supporting sustainable initiatives, reducing waste, and valuing collaborative practices are concrete ways to express a commitment to a more balanced world. Active participation in communities that promote inclusion, diversity, and social justice broadens this integrative vision, strengthening support networks and inspiring systemic change. Holism, when incorporated into everyday life, transcends the individual sphere and becomes a force for collective transformation, where every action aligned with this perspective contributes to a healthier, more compassionate, and sustainable environment. By cultivating this awareness, the journey becomes not just a quest for personal balance, but an opportunity to contribute to a future where life in all its forms can flourish fully and harmoniously.

Integrating holism into everyday life means adopting practices and attitudes that promote balance between body, mind, emotions, and spirit, allowing each aspect of existence to harmonize in a continuous flow of well-being. This balance does not happen automatically, but requires intentional choices and progressive changes, which, even if small, can have a transformative impact. Thus, living holistically involves concrete and consistent actions that sustain this broad and integrated perspective of life.

The first step on this journey is to take care of the body and health, as it is the vehicle that makes all experiences of existence possible. Eating a balanced diet, opting for natural and minimally processed foods, favors not only physical health, but also mental and emotional balance. Prioritizing nutrition rich in vegetables, fruits, whole grains, and quality proteins strengthens the body and improves disposition. In addition, maintaining a routine of physical exercise that combines aerobic activities, stretching, and muscle strengthening helps preserve vitality over the years. Adequate rest also plays an essential role, as it is during sleep that the body regenerates and the mind processes the experiences of the day. To complement this care, relaxation practices such as meditation, conscious breathing, and massage therapy help release accumulated tension, promoting a lasting feeling of well-being.

In addition to physical care, mental and intellectual development is a fundamental pillar of holism. The mind is a powerful tool for understanding and transforming reality, and therefore must be constantly nurtured with new knowledge and challenges. Reading books that expand horizons, learning new skills, and the habit of critical reflection help to avoid limited and reductionist views. Exercising creative thinking and seeking innovative solutions to everyday challenges strengthens the capacity for adaptation and resilience. Continuous learning need not be confined to formal academic settings; it can occur through the exchange of experiences with other people, the practice of hobbies that stimulate the mind, and contact with different forms of art and culture. In this way, by keeping the mind active and open, we broaden our understanding of the world and become more aware and engaged in our choices and actions.

Emotions and relationships play an essential role in the human experience, and therefore managing them intelligently is essential for a harmonious life. Practicing empathy and compassion allows us to better understand the emotions of others and strengthen genuine connections. Active listening, without judgment or interruption, strengthens interpersonal bonds and creates a safe space for dialogue. In addition, open and honest communication avoids unnecessary conflict and promotes healthier and more balanced relationships. On an individual level, learning to deal with difficult emotions such as anxiety and frustration, through techniques such as conscious breathing, journaling (therapeutic writing), and therapy, enables greater self-knowledge and emotional control. In this way, by nurturing relationships based on respect and mutual understanding, we cultivate more harmonious environments, both in personal life and in the community.

Spiritual connection and the search for transcendence are aspects that complement this holistic journey. Regardless of the belief or practice adopted, spirituality offers a space for connection with something greater, providing purpose and meaning to existence. Meditation, prayer, contemplation of nature, or even involvement with life philosophies that value self-knowledge are possible ways to nurture this dimension. Spiritual connection need not be linked to specific dogmas or religions; it can manifest itself in the simple appreciation of the beauty of the world, in the practice of gratitude, or in the perception of interdependence between all beings. By cultivating this dimension, we develop a more compassionate outlook and a greater sense of belonging to the whole.

Recognizing our interdependence with the environment and adopting sustainable practices are fundamental attitudes to living holism fully. Small daily actions, such as reducing plastic consumption, opting for ethically sourced products, and valuing the circular economy, make a big difference in environmental impact. Recycling, conscious consumption, and support for ecological initiatives are concrete ways to express respect for the planet. In addition, practices such as composting, efficient use of natural resources, and choosing sustainable means of transport significantly reduce the ecological footprint. By living more in line with nature, we strengthen the relationship between personal well-being and planetary balance.

Living holistically also involves a commitment to social and community participation. Involvement in collective projects, voluntary actions, and social initiatives strengthens community ties and extends the impact of individual transformations to the collective. Acting in groups that promote inclusion, diversity, and social justice is a way to expand awareness and contribute to a more equitable world. Civic engagement, whether through participation in community councils, social movements, or local activities, allows each individual to play an active role in building a more sustainable and harmonious future. In this way, holism ceases to be an individual practice and becomes a transformative movement that benefits the whole society.

The power of small changes should not be underestimated. Living holistically does not require radical or immediate transformations; on the contrary, it is the small daily adjustments that generate a profound and lasting impact. Setting aside a few minutes a day to practice mindfulness, observing thoughts and emotions without judgment, helps cultivate awareness of the present moment. The practice of gratitude, reflecting on positive aspects of life, strengthens emotional well-being and changes perspective on challenges. Connecting with nature regularly, whether through outdoor walks or the simple act of caring for plants, reinforces the feeling of belonging to the natural world. Valuing diversity and seeking to learn from different cultures and perspectives broadens understanding and promotes a more inclusive environment. Finally, acting with awareness and responsibility, considering the impacts of daily choices, strengthens the commitment to a more balanced lifestyle aligned with the principles of holism.

At the heart of this journey, community and collaboration play an essential role. Creating support networks that foster solidarity and cooperation strengthens social ties and offers valuable support to those seeking to live in a more integrated way. Cooperatives, community banks, and mutual support groups are examples of structures that encourage this collaboration. Promoting sustainable practices within communities, such as urban agriculture and the use of renewable energy, contributes to greater local resilience. In addition, strengthening participatory democracy through citizen assemblies and public consultations allows the community to have an active voice in building collective solutions.

Living holism in everyday life is a path of constant learning, growth, and transformation. By integrating the physical, mental, emotional, and spiritual dimensions, and by recognizing the interconnection between all life forms, we can create a more balanced and conscious reality. Holism invites us to see the world as a living and interdependent organism, where each individual choice reverberates in the collective. By embracing this perspective, we cultivate a more meaningful existence and contribute to a more just, sustainable, and harmonious future.

By adopting holism as a way of life, we realize that it does not require perfection or drastic immediate changes, but rather a continuous commitment to balance and awareness. Every small choice, from the way we eat to the way we relate to others and to the planet, contributes to a virtuous cycle of well-being and transformation. This process does not mean eliminating challenges or avoiding difficulties, but rather facing them with a more integrated perspective, seeking solutions that consider the whole instead of just isolated parts of reality.

This journey also reminds us of the importance of flexibility and adaptation. The world is constantly changing, and living holistically does not mean following rigid rules, but rather cultivating an open and curious mindset that allows for adjustments as new learning and experiences emerge. Balance is not a fixed state, but a dynamic dance between different aspects of life. Learning to listen to one's own body, mind, and emotions, respecting the natural rhythms of each phase of life, is essential to maintain this harmony.

In the end, living holism in everyday life is an act of connection - with oneself, with others, and with the world. It is an invitation to awaken the awareness that every action has an impact, that individual well-being is linked to the collective, and that true change begins within each one of us. Small gestures of presence, compassion, and respect create waves of transformation that expand beyond us, shaping a more balanced, sustainable, and humane reality. This is the true power of a life lived with intention and integration.

Epilogue

As you close these pages, a realization may have begun to settle within you—one that does not merely reside in the intellect but resonates in the very fabric of your being. Perhaps you have not merely read a book, but rather undergone a shift, an expansion, an awakening to the intricate, living tapestry of existence.

This is not the end of a journey; it is the beginning of a new way of seeing, of being, of participating in the vast and sacred dance of life. The insights contained within these pages were never meant to be confined to words, nor simply admired as abstract philosophies. They are meant to be lived.

Now, you know: the world is not a collection of isolated fragments, nor are you a separate entity adrift in an indifferent universe. You are woven into the grand design, your consciousness interlaced with all that is. Science has revealed it through quantum entanglement, ecology has demonstrated it through interdependence, and ancient traditions have whispered it for millennia: all things are connected, and within that connection, there is meaning.

What will you do with this knowledge?

For too long, humanity has operated under the illusion of separation. We have built walls—between ourselves and nature, between reason and intuition, between the personal and the collective. We have clung to reductionist paradigms, dissecting reality into parts, believing that through division, we could master understanding. But now, you have glimpsed something deeper: the universe is whole, and so are you.

Holistic thought is not an abstract concept; it is a lived experience. It is the way the rivers shape the land, the way the stars influence the tides, the way a single act of kindness ripples through the unseen fabric of existence. It is in the breath you take, drawn from the same air that has sustained every being before you. It is in the soil beneath your feet, holding the memory of all life that has ever walked upon it.

If there is a call in these pages, it is not merely to understand holism but to embody it. To walk through the world with reverence, to recognize that every action is not isolated but part of a greater unfolding. To step beyond the illusion of separateness and live in alignment with the truth that everything you think, feel, and do affects the whole.

And now, as you turn back to your own life, something will be different. Perhaps subtly at first—a pause before a decision, an awareness of an unnoticed pattern, a deeper sense of connection in moments once deemed ordinary. This is how transformation begins: not in grand gestures, but in quiet, persistent shifts in perception.

The path forward is yours to walk. You may integrate these ideas into your daily existence, allowing them to reshape your relationships, your choices, your understanding of self and world. Or you may simply carry within you the quiet knowing that you are part of something vast, something intelligent, something infinitely whole.

Either way, the journey does not end here.

The pages may close, but the understanding remains. The path continues. The interconnected web of life, of consciousness, of existence itself—welcomes you home.

www.ingramcontent.com/pod-product-compliance
Lightning Source LLC
LaVergne TN
LVHW040050080526
838202LV00045B/3574